Issues in Ethics and Applied Ethics Series

Volume-IV (Part I)

Biomedical Ethics

Issues in Ethics and Applied Ethics Series

Vol. 1	Ethics in Business, Applied and Environment
Vol. 2	Ethics in Feminism
Vol. 3	Socio-political Ethics
Vol. 4	Biomedical Ethics (Part I)
	Biomedical Ethics (Part II)
Vol. 5	Metaethics (Part I)
	Normative Ethics and Virtue Ethics (Part II)

Forthcoming volumes

Vol. 6	Ethics of Business and Economics
Vol. 7	Ethics of Charvaka/Lokayata, Morality and Secularism (Part I)
Vol. 8	Ethics of the Jainism (Part I)
Vol. 9	Ethics of the Buddhism (Part I)
Vol. 10	Ethics of Values and Education

About the Editors

Shiva Nath Prasad, after completing his studies, served Bihar Government in several capacities. After retirement he became a full timer in the pursuit of philosophy. He edited a bilingual journal *Abhranta* later edited two journals separately one in English namely Journal of Bihar Philosophical Research and *Darshan Digdarshan* in Hindi. He authored one book *Charvaka/Lokayata Analytical and Hermeneutics Study,* a very unique book, which is a "singular attempt to reconstruct this almost a vanished system of India." He also published an Anthology namely Phenomenology: Methodological Introduction with Prof. V.T. Sebastian of Panjab University. His Multi Volume Anthology on Ethics and Applied Ethics (more than fifteen volumes) are being published by Concept Publishing Company Pvt. Ltd. and some are being processed. His latest book just published is "Reflections on Charvaka/Lokayata, the Gita and Rajneesh."

Avinash Kumar Srivastava, born, December 1955 (at Village Singthu, Nalanda District, Bihar) completed Master's degree (Philosophy) from Patna University, Ph.D. on the topic "A Comparative Study of the Samadhi (Yoga) in Early Buddhism and *Bhagavad Gita*" from Magadha University, Bodh Gaya. Presently he is Professor & Head, P.G. Deptt. of Philosophy, Magadha University, P.G. Centre Darshnik Traimasik (Patna), Nalanda College Biharsharif. He is a prolific writer. He has authored two books *(Living Buddhism and Bharatiya Darshan Ki Mool Samasyayen)* and edited three Anthologies. His about fifty research papers have been published in India and abroad. He is a widely known scholar of India. He was *Joint Secretary and Secretary* of *Akhil Bharatiya Darshan Parishad and General Secretary, Bihar Darshan Parishad, Vice President of Indian Society for Buddhist Studies.* And member of editorial board of *Buddha Prajna Sindhu, and Ocean of Buddhist Wisdom (Delhi), Journal of Bihar Philosophical Research, Darshan Digdarshan (Patna).*

Issues in Ethics and Applied Ethics Series

Volume - IV (Part - I)

Biomedical Ethics

Edited by
Shiva Nath Prasad
Avinash Kumar Srivastava

CONCEPT PUBLISHING COMPANY PVT. LTD.
NEW DELHI-110059

ISBN-13: 978-81-8069-976-4 (Series)
ISBN-13: 978-93-5125-208-5 (Set)
ISBN-13: 978-81-8069-980-1 [Volume-IV (Part-I)]

First Published 2018

Published and Printed by

Concept
Since 1974

Concept Publishing Company Pvt. Ltd.
A/15-16, Commercial Block, Mohan Garden
New Delhi-110059 (India)
T: 25351460, 25351794
E: publishing@conceptpub.com, W: www.conceptpub.com

Cataloging in Publication Data--Courtesy: D.K. Agencies (P) Ltd. <docinfo@dkagencies.com>

Biomedical ethics / edited by Shiva Nath Prasad, Avinash Kumar Srivastava.
pages cm. -- (Issues in ethics and applied ethics series ; volume - IV, part I)
Includes bibliographical references and index.
ISBN 9788180699764 (Series)
ISBN 9789351252085 (Set)
ISBN 9788180699801 (Volume-IV, part I)

1. Bioethics. 2. Medical ethics. I. Prasad, Shiva Nath, editor. II. Śrīvāstava, Avināśa, 1955-, editor. III. Series: Issues in ethics and applied ethics series ; volume - IV (Part I).

DDC 174.2 23

Foreword with Comments

In the present collection of essays, Sri S.N. Prasad and Prof. Avinash Kumar Srivastava have planned to give up-to-date account of recent trends and development in Bioethics. The Anthologies on Biomedical Ethics have tried to pinpoint current issues in Applied Ethics. It will serve as a valuable text for students and teachers of Bioethics. The collection is indeed excellent and to a great extent authentic because the essays in it have been written by eminent teachers. It covers problems related to Abortion, Sexual Ethics, Euthanasia, Human Cloning, Ageing, Animal Rights, Transplantation of Human Organs, Intellectual Property Rights and Bio-Technology and Ethics. This book amply exhibits the changing trends in the field of Ethics. The book is up-to-date, because most of the essays have been written by university teachers, who are well-versed and well acquainted with the latest developments in the field of Bioethics. The Applied Ethics anticipates as to how the theory needs to be applied to solve practical moral problems. Biomedical Ethics is an important branch of Applied Ethics.

In post-modern time there is a widespread concern over moral issues in society, because of the demand for new courses on the subject of Applied Ethics, This book is quite relevant. Mr. Prasad has tried to provide overview of the Biomedical Ethics by selecting contemporary life problems.

Dr. Koeli Chakravarti and Debasri Basu are prone to subscribe to the view that some abortions are morally justified. They support the moderate view. The abortionists and anti-abortionists have conflicting views. The anti-abortionists hold that the foetus is a potential person. The conservatives believe that abortion is a kind of killing human being. Moderate view is that foetus is not human being in the early stage of pregnancy. Moral justification cannot be ascribed to the future being of the foetus, at least, in early stage. But the question is when does foetus assume the shape of person ? The question is when the foetus become a person. The Catholic Christian and Islamic fundamentalists and abortion conservative Hindus are against abortion, because abortion is ethically not justified. The concept of a person is part of moral concept. The person has a right to be treated as a member of the community. Genetic humanity is neither necessary nor sufficient to prove that an entity is a person. It is possible for a being to be genetically human and yet not be a person. Dr. Chakravarti and Dr. Basu have taken pains to consider the conservative and liberal views regarding moral status of the foetus. The moderate view is that some abortion can be morally, justified, while some cannot. Dr. Chakravarti and Dr. Basu supports moderate view. They repeat termination of unwanted pregnancies.

Here an attempt has been made by authors like Pratima Ganguli and Madhubala Kumari to deal with the problems of Euthanasia. Authors have tried to provide theoretical framework within which practical moral problems can be solved. The concern for Bioethics reflects the growing awareness of the many moral issues which beset the post-modern world. In opposition to traditional morality, a new morality seems to have emerged. Philosophers like Dr. Devarakonda Balaganapathi, Dr. R.K. Sinha and Sumit Siddharth are deeply concerned with changing attitudes towards sex and various rights movements. New problems have also been created by scientific and technological changes, including the many issues of bioethics written by Sri S.N. Prasad. It focusses on matters of foetus written by Dr. Koeli Chakravarti, Dr. Debasri Basu and Dr. M.P. Chaurasia.

New philosophical concerns have been evoked especially by a growing number of moral controversies. In traditional morality we have been largely concerned with matter of right and wrong conduct. There was an urge to do what is right ? Traditional philosophers of ethics shared beliefs about the rightness or wrongness of acts. Philosophers were mostly concerned with principles. The problem of ethics is not so much of justifying moral beliefs traditional philosophers are concerned with the theory of construction than on problems of moral application. Applied Ethics is also critical of metaethics. Analytic philosophers could not pay due attention to substantive moral issues like intellectual property rights. In fact, most metaethicists have felt, it is name of the business of philosophers to address practical issues. The emotivists for example, have taken the position that there is no such thing as moral truth. Intuitionists have argued that moral truth cannot be discovered by reason. Post-modern relativists, like Richard Rorty has claimed that morality is a matter of cultural perspectives.

But today, there are philosophers who have proposed substantive issues like human cloning and intellectual property rights. Since 1970s, moral philosophers have been addressing contemporary moral issues like Ageing and Animal Rights. Peter Singer in his book *Applied Ethics* have dealt with Abortion, Animals Right and Euthanasia. Thus, new fields of Applied Ethics have developed. They have provided new models for making practical decisions and resolving disputes. Contemporary Indian philosophers do have something to offer in the field of Bioethics. They have tried to apply theories into concrete Bioethical problems like abortion and cloning some of the critics uphold that there is still a gap between Theoretical and Applied Ethics. The reason for criticism is due to the fact that the work in Applied Ethics presupposes the position of one or another schools of moral philosophy. The other criticism is that Applied Ethics is done without any explicit attention to theory at all.

The discussion on sexual morality gained relevance especially in the context of the rise of HIV/AIDS. Dr. Devarakonda Balaganapathi upholds that trust and responsibility in the sexual morality in the context of HIV/AIDS are important. He argues that only in a single partner, known and long term relationship trust and responsibility are strong and hence only by adopting such a relationship, it is possible to avoid transmission of AIDS. Trust requires mutual understanding. To be responsible for something is to be answerable for it. A responsible person discharges his responsibilities. It can be understood that whenever there is trust, there ought to be responsibility and wherever there is responsibility, trust would definitely exist there. Trust and responsibility are two sides of any relationship. Mistrust and irresponsibility would make the life of a person miserable by destroying all social relations. I feel rampant growth of AIDS has necessitated the need to look at the sexual morality afresh.

Dr. Pratima Ganguli has tried to streamline the problem of Euthanasia and its moral implications she holds that Euthanasia is neither suicide nor murder but it is denoted by 'Mercy Killing'. There is a distinction between 'Mercy Killing' and 'Mercy Death'. Mercy killing is involuntary or does not involve the patient's permission or request, whereas 'mercy death' is done with the permission of the patient. Terminally ill people may desire voluntary Euthanasia, when a person does not give his consent to die but well wishers desire to prevent unbearable suffering on the part of the person killed. There is third kind of euthanasia known as non voluntary. If person is in comma since long and is not capable to choose between life and death, euthanasia will neither be voluntary nor involuntary but non-voluntary. The question of euthanasia form an important part of Biomedical Ethics. Biomedical Ethics is a branch of Applied Ethics. The question is whether the Euthanasia is morally justified or not. Philosophers on this issue are divided in two groups, e.g., conservative and liberal. Liberals hold that it is right and it is freedom of the person whether he wants to live or die. If the person desires death in terminal case then it is not a crime. If we kill terminally ill cancer patient at his request then it will be based on mercy. Dr. Ganguli is of opinion that "if mercy death is to be allowed, there should be a guarantee that it would be morally and legally permissible". Dr. Shiva Bhanu Singh has very correctly tried to understand Euthanasia as a practice of terminating the life of a person in a painless or minimally painful way in order to stop suffering. He observes that euthanasia is a controversial issue because of conflicting moral feelings. Dr. Shiva Bhanu Singh adheres that taking one's own life is not always sin. In special circumstances cessation of life can be supported as far as the justification of voluntary euthanasia is concerned being well thought rational decision of a self conscious autonomous human being, it can be justified with certain conditions. *Cloning : Some Ethical Issues* by Dr. Jyotish Ch. Basak holds that the application of genetic cloning for the understanding and control of disease that is, therapeutic cloning is for the well-being of mankind. In 1978, the world for the first time listened to the news of the first test tube baby. Human cloning is the creation of a human being or a number of human beings, who are genetically identical to donor usually hear cloning referred to in one of two ways First, reproductive cloning, and secondly, therapeutic. cloning. Reproductive cloning refers to the creation of a new person with the same genetic make up as someone who is alive or has lived. Therapeutic cloning refers to using cloning techniques to initiate the growth of embryos in order to create new organs or cells for medical and research purpose. Cloning seems to offer new possibilities of medical advances. The Catholic Church John Pal II condemned the cloning of all life forms. Human cloning is illegal in many countries. Hillary Putnam argues that cloning human violates human dignity. Putnam is of the view that there may be misuse of cloning technology. Putnam conceives some moral images of the family. We do use images derived from family life in structuring our whole way of looking at society and our whole way of seeing our moral responsibilities to one another. We live in a moral community defined by certain basic moral concepts and principles. The question of good and bad technology cannot be decided in isolation from the question whether it seriously undermines our moral image of the world.

In the paper entitled "Human Cloning : Some Bioethical Questions" Dr. D.N. Tiwari holds that technology has almost become the synonyms of our entire advancement influencing way of life and the life style of the people of the millennium. Dr. Tiwari has pinpointed very ably about the Human Cloning in our Indian scriptures. He observes, "In *Skandha, Adhyaya* 13, of Srimad Bhagvat it has been mentioned that when his Excellency Nimi was dead, the seers by process of Mantha, perhaps human cloning in modern idioms, of his body created a new baby. The baby was called Janaka, as it was a birth out of cell of his father. It was called Videha, as it was not born from a mother but out of a non sexual, non conjugal process. As the baby was born out a process of Mantha, it was called 'Mithila' and his kingdom was named Mithila" Dr. Tiwari holds that the morality in society will also be divided into the morality of the clones and that of the rest. The clones, like Friedrich Nietzsche's superman, may claim that the utmost duty of the society is to rear clones who only have the right to live on earth. The morality of the clones based on the idea that "all that proceeds from the power is good and all that springs from weakness is bad" will upset the moral aim of equality and peace in the society. Dr. Tiwari has attempted to consider the ethics of bio technology and the morality of the Bio technologicians and Bio engineers involved in cloning. He upholds, in the end that their task of cloning cannot be termed immoral.

Ageing : A New Look' by M.P. Chaurasia upholds that we can say that even today science is in process of searching and what it has been searched out is not free from defects. From this point of view the solution forwarded by *yoga* is the best, because it follows the natural process through which one can develop resistance power of the body to fight against ageing in a natural way, Sri S.N. Prasad in his article "Ageing : A Psycho-Physiological Study : A Search from Cause to Cure" adheres that Ageing is a natural process. The old age presents a pitiable spectacle, which moved Buddha to go for *tapas*. Sri Prasad has very pertinently raised the question whether ageing is an ethical problem ? Sri Prasad has observed that 'old age is a multifaced alienation. Old age is a state of powerlessness, normlessness, isolation and meaninglessness, Powerlessness is a stage or means or refers to a stage, which makes the individual feel that he has no authority, or say in any of the matters. Normlessness creates the feeling that the social roles, standards or values are no more observed. Isolation is a stage where the individual happens to feel that he is all alone and there is none who come to his aid and listen to him. Meaninglessness is a stage where the individual feels that his existence is of no use and he has no utilitarian value for society. He mentions that in India and Japan old man is not meaningless and valueless. In India there is deep feelings and reverence for the old people. The respect for a person is a value. Immanuel Kant, the most influential German philosopher of the modern time, in his *Groundwork for a Metaphysics of Morals* puts person at the centre of morality. He argues that treating person merely as a means to our own ends is immoral. To be a person he is to be an autonomous being.

In the article entitled "Animal Rights : Ethical Perspective" by Dr. Devarakonda Balaganapathi subscribes to the moral rights of animals. In the book entitled, *Animal liberation*, The Australian Philosopher Peter Singer contends that "All animals are equal". He argued that though our shared morality protects human animals from innumerable kinds of treatment we find intolerable, it is for less protective of non-human animals and hence it is only partial Since Singer brings non-human animals also under the moral framework by following the utilitarian principle that since we morally ought to maximize happiness and minimize sufferings and as animals also can suffer, our calculations ought to include them as well. Since non-human animals, like human animals also can experience both pleasure and pain, 'if it is wrong to cause human suffering to achieve a good that does not outweigh that suffering then it is wrong to cause non-human suffering to achieve a good'.

Again the article entitled "Morality of Human Sexuality" by Dr. M.P. Chaurasia emphasizes that sex is an essential phenomenon, not only of human beings but also of animals and insects. But sexual relationship of animal are beyond the purview of moral judgments. The sexual activities of human beings come under the purview of moral consideration because their actions affect others. As per recent trends perhaps people who believe is traditional values are considered Conservatives. They consider moral values as 'absolute' and think that sexual freedom is a violation of this value, which is part and parcel of our Indo Aryan heritage. Sexual activities should take place only between legally married couple. All kinds of rapes, child molestation and sadism are considered wholly immoral. All sexual activities performed between the consenting adults are moral as long as it cannot harm others.

The article entitled Bioethics and the Buddha by Prof. Angraj Chaudhary attempts to emphasize that Buddha regarded man as the greatest of all beings. Man alone can practice *Dhamma* and attain *Nirvana*. Dr. Chaudhary states that medical researchers who make experiments on animals in order to discover suitable and efficacious medicines for mankind cannot be ethically blamed because their intention is not to take their life. Medicines they discover save precious human lives. So the intention of medical researchers being pure they are not ethically blameworthy. It is true that one of the most important five ethical percepts is to abstain from killing, but it must be remembered that he did not prescribe it for all. When soldiers fight in the war in order to defend their country from enemies, they are bound to kill and the Buddha considered it the bounded duty of the soldiers to fight and kill enemies. Buddha knew that performing different duties is essential for making a society stable. Further his article entitled "Buddha's views on Transplantation of Human organs is a very relevant one. Any ethics or ethical code in order to be universal has to face the challenges of changing time and not become irrelevant. Buddha's ethical technique stand the test of the time. It is true that Buddha does not say anything directly on transplantation of human organs. There came no occasion in his life when he was faced with such a problem. There was no so much of biomedical research in his time nor 'could the doctors of his time ever think of replacing any damaged human organs by another human organs. The well known doctor Jivak-Buddha's personal physician could perform miraculous surgery but there is no reference to transplantation of human organ. This is a contribution of modern science and modern bio medical research. Dr. Chaudhary has observed, "I do not think the Buddha could ever have raised any objection to the transplantation of human organs, if by doing so a precious human life could be saved". By transplanting kidney, Doctor saves a precious human life. If we read between the lines of some of the passages in the *Tripitaka* it will be clear that man according to Buddha occupies a higher place in the hierarchy of beings. It is man who can become Buddha. Buddhism and Jainism both believe is non-violence. The difference is that Buddhism is liberal whereas Jainism follows it in letter and spirit. Dr. Choudhary observes, "I think Itsing, the Chinese traveller, succinctly expresses the Buddha's" view of non-violence when he says that, 'if man will protect each and every being he will himself become unprotected and will have to lose his life for nothing".

Prof Nirbhai Singh's aritcle entitled 'Bioethics and Indian Culture' purports to focus attention on bioethics and Indian culture. The concept of bioethics is a new branch of ethics which has come up in the philosophical circles. It focusses on ethical aspects of life for improving upon moral quality of life in society. It makes doctors of their more obligation. It takes up vital social issues. Bioethics is an attempt for healing the ailing humans.

The article entitled 'Intellectual Property Rights : A Bird's Eye View, by Dr. Rakesh Kumar Sinha has tried to present a new ethical dimension relating to Intellectual Property Rights. As a matter of fact Intellectual Property refers to creations of the mind. Dr. Rakesh has considered the division of Intellectual Property into two categories. Industrial property, which includes inventions (patents), trade marks, industrial design, and geographic indications of source, layout designs of integrated circuit and copyright, which includes literary and artistic words such as drawing, paintings, photographs and sculptures, and architectural designs.

The basic obligation in the area of patents is that, invention in all branches of technology whether products or process shall be patentable if they meet the three tests of being new, involving an inventive step and being capable of industrial application. Today a patent is an exclusive right awarded to an inventor to prevent others from making, selling, distributing, importing, or using their invention, without licence or authorisation, for a fixed period of time.

The chapter entitled "Intellectual Property" by Sumit Siddharth says that intellectual property relates to Industrial property. It includes inventions, trade marks, industrial designs and geographic indications of source whereas copy right emphasises on literary and artistic works such as novels, poems and plays, films, musical works, drawings, paintings, photographics, sculptures and architectural designs.

Intellectual property is the legal characterization of biotechnological process example transformed microorganisms, developed improved varieties, etc. Intellectual property protection (IPP) and Intellectual Property Rights (IPR) are available to protect this property. According to Sumit, Intellectual property is an abstract property against tangible (real) physical property which one can feel, see and use in physical forms.

Dr. Madhubala Kumari has tried to define euthanasia as an action in which a person is allowed to die because it is believed that the individual would be better off dead than alive. Hence, euthanasia is painless death of a person who is suffering a terminal or incurable disease. Mercy killing is a good death. The purpose is to end the suffering. In conclusion, Dr. Madhubala says that in spite of the great diversity of views, we can say that the practice of Euthanasia should be allowed on certain critical circumstances when all hopes of his life or her life has gone off.

The essay on 'No Flesh Eating : Buddhist Perspective of Vegeterianism, by Dr. Avinash Kumar Srivastava presents some complex ethical principles that have been discussed down the ages. Dr. Srivastava has streamlined its importance in the present world. Vegetarianism means to support ones life on grains, fruits, milk, cereals, and vegetables only and not to take flesh in any form. In the present world, the need for vegetarian food is emphasized for two reasons. First, the pragmatic. reason is to avoid merciless killing of animals which has caused great problem to our ecology. The second reason is concerned with human health and hygiene. It is evident that regular flesh eating causes diseases. Physicians have started prescribing vegetarian food. Dr. Srivastava has approached the problem from the perspectives of Buddhist ethics. '*Panatipata* veramani' is the watchword of Buddhist ethics. Buddhists adhere to the precept of non killing and observe, '*Samma Ajiva*'. As a matter of fact, Buddha neither prescribed vegetarianism nor recommended flesh eating. His teaching of non violence implies no flesh eating because flesh eating involves violence towards animal. Flesh eating is not in tune with Buddhist Philosophy.

The paper of Madhumita Chaterjee presents a good proper on Bioethics.

The article entitled "Health : A Positive Bioethical concept underlying *vinayapitaka* by Riddhi Chakravarty attempts to explore the relation between bioethics and health. Buddhism upholds holistic model of health. The author has also tried to explicate the concept of health as found in the test of *vinaypitak*. In nutshell, the author has tried to establish that the concept of health has been a recent bioethical concern but Buddhism had propounded the concept much earlier. Buddhism propounded the concept of positive health. This perspective of health in Buddhism can be said in one sense to reflect the recent concern of bioethics.

The book entitled *Biomedical Ethics* presents a detailed account of problems of Biomedical ethics. It is certainly a significant addition to works on Applied Ethics. I welcome the book. The first distinguishing feature of the work lies in the way it situates its task in the face of normative and metaethics. The strength of the volume lies in Prasad's efforts in identifying the problems of Bioethics. Here distinguished authors have made an attempt to apply ethical principles in the field of Bioethics. Authors have clearly demonstrated a great understanding of Bioethical problems. Contemporary Indian authors of this volume are sensitive to the problem of Bioethics and go a long way in making this Anthology important to any study of Applied Ethics. It also opens new frontiers in the arena of ongoing ethical debates. I intend to say that Bioethics constitutes an important part of Applied Ethics. Many Western schools think that Indian scholars are confined to construct philosophical scholars and neglect the problems of Bioethics. This myth has been exploded with the appearance of this book entitled *Biomedical Ethics* compiled and edited by Sri Shiva Nath Prasad. It also rejects the myth that philosophers of India over the last two thousand years have been consistently concerned with the problems of metaphysics, logic, epistemology and soteriology. My intention is not to belittle the achievements in the sphere of logic, epistemology and ontology. I admit that the contributions of Indian thinkers in the fields of Applied Ethics in general and Bioethics in particular seem to be poor indeed when viewed against their European counterparts. But the appearance book rejects my misgivings. The criticism is often raised against Indian philosophy in general that it turns its back on all theoretical and practical considerations of morality. *I think that this book refutes many misgivings about contemporary professional philosophers of India. I welcome this work as a landmark achievement in the field of Applied Ethics.*

R.C. Sinha
Retd., Head Deptt. of Philosophy,
Patna University,
Patna & Senior Research
Fellow, ICPR, Delhi

Preface

Though quite unconservatively indeed, before saying anything regarding substance and materials of the present book, first and foremost, we humbly beg to state that we falter, beg and pine for an adequate word to express our myriad and mammoth sense of gratitude to Prof. R.C. Sinha, a scholar, a visionary, a mendicant of philosophy, for whom philosophy is not a profession any longer, (retired as he is, since some years past) philosophy is not a recourse to his earning and possession, not even a pastime, since pastime is just a casual affair for whiling away time, but for him, philosophy is a passion, with limitless ardent zeal, every part of his body is filled with *elanvital* of Philosophy, as a scholar, as a visionary, as a mendicant in philosophy, travelling and touring through the country and abroad, picking and collecting nectar, ambrosia from each nook and corner from the trees of wisdom, the universities, the academia and then imparting and distributing to each and sundry, who craves for wisdom, since philosophical wisdom is the सर्व विद्या प्रतिष्ठा making it interdisciplinary, multidimensional and broad-based in every sense of the term, his tireless and relentless zeal surpass all expressions in letter and spirit.

Prof. Sinha, by writing not only a stereotyped foreword, but a detailed and lively commentary on all the papers collected in the present volume, has really eased the job and responsibility which is universally considered as essential for the editor (author) he has reduced the editor's job a big blank, a zero. Any attempt at elaboration in this regard would amount to mere cudgeling of brain over spilt milk, or mere repetition, incurring vexations, on the part of the readers worth indignation, displeasure and drudgery. So editor(s) beg the readers to excuse for not writing any thing on the contents of the papers.

Suffice it to say, that the present volume forms a part of our ambitions multi-volume series enterprise in Ethics and Applied Ethics, which would cover a vast array of ethical topics, discussed incisively by the specialist scholars of India on Ethics, each volume covering more than 300 pages approximately or even more. They will cover lot of topic which would provide interesting readings to the general curious readers, the teachers, professors, teaching philosophical ethics in the universities of India, as a matter of and part of university syllabi in ethics. The study of ethics has been necessitated and considered invincible today, more than any subject in the university syllabi as forming part of inculcating values in life, owing to the fact that due to incessant degradation of values in life, which have given place to animosities, bitterness, separateness, angularities that have been too deeply ingrained in human beings. In order to bring humaneness and humanity, humanism. The ethical reading provided in the different volumes of this series would go a long way to reconsider gravely upon the human values and inculcate values to make life an ideal life, rid of animality and bestiality.

The editors are deeply indebted to Prof. Debashish Guha, who inspired us to make fresh endeavours to concentrate on ethics, metaethics, applied ethics, which were limited to university syllabi in our student days. Due to his guidance and effort, it has become possible to concentrate on a multi-volume enterprise on ethical topics, instead of publishing one special issue of our Journal of Philosophy on Ethics and Applied Ethics.

The editors are too much thankful and obliged to all the scholars who have taken pains to send their papers for the volumes by way of cooperation in achieving academic goals.

The editors express deep regrets for the delay in the publication of the contributor's papers and praise them for keeping extreme patience during all these periods and we also beg apology on this account.

Our thanks specially go to Shri Ashok Kumar Mittalji, Concept Publishing Company Pvt. Ltd., New Delhi for consenting to publish multi-volume project on ethics and applied ethics and devoting so much of his precious time and money in the interest of people at large, and also in the interest of the post graduate students, teachers teaching philosophy, ethics, in the universities as aid material.

We are thankful to Sri Shailesh Kr. Sinha who has laboured hard in getting hand written manuscript computer typed with too much of patience. He has been a great asset in so far as typing more than thousand pages approximately, constituting four or five books.

The present book is a twenty two chaptered book, all well-knit and giving profusely clear account of the various topics in the sphere of a particular branch of philosophy, collected at one place, a newer field of practical ethics, which goes by the name of Biomedical Ethics. They provide a pleasant reading as well as afford useful substantial guide to the post graduate philosophy students, besides facilitating the teachers in teaching.

The book is in the hands of the scholars and readers and it is left to them to decide how far we have fared well or not and feel free to accept whatever appeals to them and reject what they feel they are worthy of rejection. Any discrepancy and any fault in this adventurous academic enterprise is that of the editors. But whatever the faults, they may be brought to the notice of the editors for correction, amendment in near future in the next editions. "To err is human" is the popular saying and so the editors should always be amenable to corrections.

If this book goes to serve even a bit of academic interests (in filling up the gaps of knowledge in the field of ethics) the editors would feel, they have been profoundly rewarded.

S.N. Prasad
A.K. Srivastava

Acknowledgements

The persent volume is the fourth volume from amongst the multi-volume anthologies, under the series "Issues in Ethics & Applied Ethics" and is directed to the study of Biomedical Ethics only.

It may be mentioned at the very out set, that we had started to work in the fields of ethics and applied ethics at the inspiration of Prof. Debashis Guha, who had been working in this particular field of ethics, from the very beginning and has great gained name and fame. He was then in Ranchi University, Jharkhand State. He is now Prof. in Allahabad University (U.P.). By way of a helping hand in our new venture on ethics, he not only sent several of his own specialized papers, but had also made me available, many of papers of his research scholars who completed their research in different aspects of ethics, under his able guidance. With this, we invited papers from other scholars of different universities of India. Papers soon swelled, which made all through interested in Indian philosophy, but with lots of papers which were accumulated, I contacted several Publishers. We saw that some of the books written by Prof. Guha, had been published by M/s Concept Publishing Company Pvt. Ltd., New Delhi. We also contacted the Proprietor of Concept Publishing Company Pvt. Ltd., New Delhi. With heavy support, help, cooperation and encouragement of the scholars specialized in the field of ethics, our original plan for two or three volumes anthology in ethics has almost swelled now to more than twenty volumes. We are still encouraged for more volumes, if time and life permit. Since ethics is not one day affair, we need it every day, every moment. Every time, we are confronted with new ethical problems, which we need to redress; we need more and more ethics, and still more; as hard times come and enhance mental pressure and affect all and sundry, every one wishes to get through the ordeals of trial and tribulations. These are natural tendencies of all human beings.

In spite of all the helps and encouragements we were having from the scholars, what remained biting our conscience was over the inordinate delay in the publication of the papers of the scholar which exceeded lots of years. We feel enormous guilt of conscience for this and no word of apology can be sufficient for them. Even this day ie this day we are writing. This note is not the end of their period of anxious awaiting. It may take still some more months, for the contributing scholars to have their books in their hands, we once again pray them, to grant us some more time, with still more apologies from us. We have expressed our humble submission to the Proprietor of M/s Concept Publishing Company Pvt. Ltd., New Delhi for speedy completion and rid us from this agony.

We are very much thankful to Sri S.K. Sinha and Anil Kumar Sinha who have computer typed hand wtitten papers with much of patience and painstaking. We have still more typed materials for publications.

In the end, we thank Shri Ashok Kumar Mittal, Concept Publishing Company Pvt. Ltd., New Delhi, to agree to publish our multi-volume anthologies with keen interest, keeping in his mind the larger benefits and interests of the research scholars, students as well as general readers and the teachers of this important field of knowledge. We have interest in human values, for the happiness of human community, so to say, for the sake of common unity. Let us all join in this great HUMAN ENTERPRISE.

Shiva Nath Prasad

Avinash Kumar Srivastava

Contents

List of Contributors

Prof. Koeli Chakravarti, Retd., Prof. Deptt. of Philosophy, University of Burdwan (West Bengal).

Prof. Debasri Basu, University of Burdwan, West Bengal.

Dr. Devarakonda Balaganapathi, Deptt. of Philosophy, Dravidian University, Kuppam-517425. *Email-balaganapathid @rediffmail.com*

Prof. Pratima Ganguli, Deptt. of Philosophy, (Retd.). Bhagalpur University, Bihar.

Dr. Shiva Bhanu Singh, Deptt. of Philosophy, Ewing Chirstian College, Allahabad, (U.P.).

Dr. Jyotish Chandra Basak, Deptt., of Philosophy, North Hill University, Shillong (Maghalaya)

Prof. D.N. Tiwari, Prof. and Head, Deptt. of Philosophy, Banaras Hindu University, Varanasi, (U.P.).

Prof. Angraj Chaudhary, Retd. Prof., a great Buddhist scholar, Recipient of President Award.

Prof. Nirbhai Singh, Retd. Prof., Panjabi University, Patiala, Member I.C.P.R. Delhi.

Rakesh Kumar Sinha, Senior Scientist Officer, Delhi.

Sumit Siddharth, Research Scholar in Bio-Technology, Kalinga University, Bhubaneswar (Odisha).

Dr. Madhubala Kumari, Head, Deptt. of Philosophy, Islamia College, Siwan, Bihar.

Dr. Madhumita Chatterjee, C-8/1, Chirantune Park, Bansadroni, Kolkata (WB).

M.P. Chaurasia, Deptt. of Philosophy, J.P. University, Chapra (Saran), (Bihar).

Prof. Avinash Kumar Srivastava, Magadha University, Bodh Gaya (Nalanda College), Biharshariff (Bihar).

Ms. Riddhi Chakravarty, Research Scholar, Deptt. of Humanities and Social Sciences, I.I.T. Kharagpur-721302 (W.B.).

Prof. Sinha, R.C., S.R. Fellow-ICPR, (W.B).

Shiva Nath Prasad, Road No. 20, Plot No. 39, S.K. Nagar, Patna-800001 (Bihar).

Email: shivanathprasad51@yahoo.com

Chapter 1

The Moral Status of the Foetus

Koeli Chakravarti & Debasri Basu

Abortion is a highly controversial issue. Thinkers have fought bitterly against one another over this issue. Sometimes pro-abortion arguments have got upper hand. At other times anti-abortion argument have gained stronger ground. In this Chapter we will be concerned with one of the crucial questions around which the abortion debate revolves. The question is about the moral status of the foetus, Does the foetus have any rights? The abortionist and the anti-abortionist have different answers to offer. The view which holds that abortion is never ethically acceptable is the conservative view, while the view which considers abortion to be ethically acceptable at any point of foetus development is the view of the liberals. The third view is the moderate view which considers abortion to be permissible up to a certain point of foetal development. According to the *conservatives* the foetus enjoys a full moral status. The liberals on the other hand do not consider the foetus to have any significant moral status. Those who hold the *moderate* view think that the foetus has only a partial moral status.

The prominent conservative view is mainly associated with the Roman Catholic Church which forbids direct killing of innocent human life. The opponents of abortion think that it is a person or a human being that we kill when we abort. There are two kinds of claim on which the case against abortion usually rests. One claim is that the *foetus is a human being or a potential person.*

The claim that the foetus is a human being is often put forward as follows. The conservatives believe that there is a continuum between a zygote and a child, and that abortion is equivalent to killing a person or human being. No discrimination, the conservatives insists should be made among human beings on grounds of the different potentialities they might have. If one is conceived by human parents, and thus has a human genetic code, one ought to be treated as a human being. To the conservatives, conception is the moment at which one starts being a person, since it is during conception that the genetic endowments of the future adult are fused into one unit. The conservatives thus make conception the boundary between the non-human and human.

There is indeed a sense in which the claim that the foetus is a human being can be said to be a legitimate claim. The foetus is undeniably a member of our species rather than any of any other. The very fact that we admit that the foetus is already a member of our species would imply that that species is certainly our species. But that simply amounts to begging the question because that is precisely the issue that is in dispute. The question around which the controversy has developed is whether the foetus is so developed as to be regarded as a member of any species at all.

Any one who approaches the problem of abortion by claiming that the foetus is a human being has to face a major objection which is sometimes described as the boundary problem[1] i.e., the problem regarding the precise boundary between a foetus and a human being. What is the *exact line of demarcation* between a foetus and human being? At what point in the continuous line of development of the foetus does a 'human life emerge'?

There is another objection that anyone who claims that the foetus is a human being has to answer. This claim can stand only if we appeal to its potential rather than to its actual properties. Anyone who says that the foetus has a stronger claim to life than animals has to justify himself by appealing to morally relevant properties, and this can only be done in terms of the potential of the foetus. But to claim that the foetus is a potential human being is to put forward a different argument altogether.

We now come to the second claim, the claim that the foetus has all the potentialities of a person. This argument suggests that what we really value and want to preserve is the future being of the foetus. This amounts to saying that abortion is wrong because it destroys the life of a person who would have existed in future. But the same argument, as Glover points out, can be advanced against contraception. Glover points out that those who oppose both abortion and contraception tend to consider abortion to morally worse than contraception. The argument behind claim, that abortion is a greater evil than contraception is that in the case of abortion the life of the foetus as a potential person has already started while contraception tries to prevent the very inception of life.The weakness of the argument lies in the fact that it does not explain why termination of the process is worse at one state or another when our main interest lies in not losing the person who is being developed and who will come out at the end of the process. The argument cannot explain why abortion is worse than contraception until it considers the stage of development to be an important, the argument is no longer the same; but has shifted from potentiality to actuality from the properties of the person the foetus may become to the properties the foetus now has. So the question that now has to be answered is when does one become a person?

We have pointed out above that various attempts have been made to find a dividing line between a foetus and a child. Of these different attempts we have already discussed the one that considers conception to be the dividing line. Let us note, consider the other answers that have been put forward.

Some consider birth to be the dividing line, some think that it is viability that should be the boundary, while some others think that quickening or the first movement of the foetus marks the dividing line. It is not difficult to understand why birth is suggested as the time when a foetus becomes a person. It is only after a baby is born that he or she is accepted into the human community. It is also at birth that the child can express his or her distinctive personality. The conservatives, however, think that birth cannot decide whether or not a being may be killed. They believe that the foetus is the same entity, whether it is inside the mother's body or outside it. It has the same human characteristics (whether we see them or not), the same sensitivity and the same degree of awareness. A prematurely born infant may be less developed than a full term foetus, but to the pro-abortionists, it is wrong to kill the latter. Those who oppose abortion fail to understand why the mere location of a being can make such a difference to the wrongness of killing it.

Viability of the foetus is often considered to be the point when the foetus becomes a person. The point when a baby is capable of surviving without depending on others is considered to be of tremendous importance. It is the time when it becomes a potentially independent creature for the first time. The argument for viability has to answer two objections.[2] First, on this account potential physical independence is regarded as a necessary condition of being a person. But it may so happen that with improved technology a very old person is kept alive by making him or her dependent on another person's body. The old person then would not be regarded as viable, but would certainly be recognized as a person. The argument for viability, therefore, should explain why viability is considered to be the dividing line at one end of life alone, and not at the other end as well. The second objection runs as follows. The argument for viability has to recognize the fact that viability is not a fixed boundary but is liable to shift. Twenty-eight weeks is generally considered to be the time when a foetus begins to be viable, but such a sharp boundary line cannot always be drawn. Many babies are not viable even when they are born earlier.

Another problem with the argument for viability is found to vary with the state of medical technology.[3] Thirty years ago, a premature baby born two months before the due date could not easily survive, but these days with improved medical technology even a six month old foetus can survive. Whether or not a premature baby will survive also depends on the place where the baby is born. Chances of survival are higher if the place of birth is a big city having good medical facilities. The abortionists believe that the foetus cannot be granted right to life independent of the wishes of its mother because it is to its mother that it owes its survival. To the anti-abortionists it is wrong to argue in this way because a person's life may depend totally on another and yet nobody would think that the latter has the right to decide whether or not the former will continue to live. A son does not have the right to decide whether or not his elderly mother would live simply in view of the fact that she totally depends on him. Similarly, a non-viable foetus may depend on its mother but that does not mean that the mother has a right to put an end to its life.

The first movement of the foetus felt by an expectant mother is known as quickening and is something considered to be another dividing line between the foetus and the child. Traditional Christian theology believed that it is at this moment that the foetus was endowed with a soul, the possession of soul being the distinguishing mark of man. Contemporary Catholic theologians, however, no longer think that the foetus gains its soul at the time it first starts moving. The argument thus loses its significance for the first time. It is true that the capacity of the foetus to move develops at a particular time, but that does not mean that other people would make judgements regarding its right to live. When people become paralysed they cannot walk any more but they do not thereby lose their right to life.

The real dispute between the abortionists and the anti-abortionists is a dispute about the time when a foetus becomes a human being. The anti-abortionists believe that it is difficult to find a morally significant dividing line between the foetus and the new born baby, that the development of a human being from a zygote is a thoroughly gradual process. If there is no dividing line between a zygote and a child, two possible lines of action may be taken either the status of the zygote will be upgraded to that of the child, or the status of the child will be downgraded to that of the zygote. But nobody thinks that children should be 'dispatched' as and when their parents request. Hence the only justifiable line of action, the conservatives point out, is to protect the foetus just as we protect the child.

We have seen above that various attempts have been made to find an answer to the question: when does one become a person? There is, however a certain arbitrariness in attempting to draw sharp boundaries like conception, birth, viability etc.[4] There are two ways in which this attempt may be shown to be arbitrary. First, 'person' is a loose concept. As Glover points out, it is not easy to draw a satisfactory line round the concept of person. We cannot single out one particular feature as constituting personhood. Instead there is a cluster of different features, such as, being conscious, being able to respond emotionally and so on. Moreover, even if personhood stands for a whole cluster of various characteristics, it would be wrong to think that all such characteristics develop at the same time or at the same rate.

The second reason why it is arbitrary to draw sharp boundaries is that the transition from a fertilised ovum to a grown up person is a biological development, and like so many biological developments should be represented by more or less gradual upward curve rather than by a series of sharply different stages marked by sudden changes. One is not promoted to the status of a person on one particular day. Just as childhood, youth, middle age or old age does not begin on one specific date, so also there is no one particular date on which one attains personhood. We can indeed fix up specific age boundaries for legal or social purposes. For example, in many countries eighteen is considered the age when one ceases to be a minor and become a major. But this is largely a convention and not a reflection of the biological reality.

Becoming a person is thus a gradual process, a matter of degree. Glover admits that this approach does not solve all difficulties because one might still disagree regarding the time when the process of increasing personalisation begins or ends. The only redeeming feature is that these disagreements are not factual but are disagreements regarding the importance of different degrees of development. Hence, they are not strong enough to refute the contention that becoming a person has a gradual ascending slope.

Let us now take a look at the liberal standpoint regarding the moral status of the foetus. The foetus, liberals generally believe, continues to remain non-human even when it reaches the most advanced stages of development. The liberals do not deny that a foetus is a human being from the biological point of view. The point that they want to make is that the foetus is not human in any morally significant sense. A lucid discussion of this approach can be found in *Mary Anne, Warren's article 'On the Moral and Legal Status of Abortion'*[5] Warren draws a distinction between two senses of the term 'human': the *genetic sense* and the *moral sense.* In the genetic sense any member of the species Homo Sapiens is a human being, members of no other species can be human in this sense. An individual can be said to be human in the moral sense when he or she is a 'full-fledged member of the moral community'. Warren says that whatever is genetically human, need not also be morally human. A moral community, according to Warren, is one that consists of person only, rather than genetically human beings.

Warren considers the following characteristics to be basic to be concept of personhood. (1) Consciousness, and particularly the capacity to feel pain; (2) Capacity to reason, that enables one to solve new and complex problems; (3) Self-motivated activity, (4) The capacity to communicate and indefinite variety of things in different ways; (5) The capacity to form concepts about oneself.

If a being does not satisfy any of these five conditions, he or she is definitely not a person. Warren rightly points out that the concept of a person is in part a moral concept. To recognise someone as a person is to admit that the person has a right to be treated as a member of the moral community. Genetic humanity is neither necessary nor sufficient to prove that an entity is a person. It is possible for a being to be genetically human, and yet not be a person. When a man or a woman continues to live with permanently impaired consciousness, we say that he or she continues to live, not as a person but as a human being. A foetus too is a human being, but it is yet to develop as a person, and does not have full moral rights.

The question that needs to be asked at this point is: Is it proper to say that a foetus does not have a right to life just because it is not a full-fledged member of the moral community? Anti-abortionists believe that even if a foetus does not have full-fledged moral rights and is not fully a person as yet, it is still (i) Like a person, and (ii) has the potential for becoming a person, and thus has a right to life.

Let us see what liberals have to say with regard to these contentious issues. Warren admits that living being resembling persons but not fulfilling the requirements of personhood may have moral rights, but the more person like a being is the stronger reasons does it have for claiming a right to life, and the stronger its right to life is. Thus if there is a continuity in the biological development of the human individual, there will be a similar continuity in the development of his or her moral rights. At the same time, what needs to be noted is that the attributes which decide whether or not a being is enough like a person to be regarded as having some of the same moral rights are the same as those which decide whether or not a being is fully a person. They are not different from the five conditions of personhood mentioned above. Genetic humanity or possession of human physical features or the capacity to survive outside the mother's body are not among these relevant attributes. Hence even if a foetus in an advanced stage arouses in us as powerful a protective instinct as is generally aroused by a small infant, it is as unlike a person as a small embryo is. Warren further says that although the foetus has sensitivity to pain and a rudimentary form of consciousness, yet it is not conscious in the way a few months old infant is and does not fulfil the woman's right to have an abortion at any stage of her pregnancy.

We have so far considered the conservative and liberal views regarding the moral status of the foetus. Let us now consider the moderate view. Proponents of the moderate view believe that some abortions can be morally justified, while some cannot. Some moderates think that the stage of foetal development is a factor that one has to take into account in considering the rightness or wrongness of abortion. Some moderates are of the opinion that there are various reasons that have to be kept in mind in considering the justifiability of abortion. There are still other moderated who think that both the stage of development and the justifying reasons have to be taken into account in considering the rightness or wrongness of abortion.

Four kinds of moderate views can be found in discussions on abortion. The first view may be regarded as the moderation of the conservative standpoint. Like the conservatives, the moderates of this group believe that the foetus has full moral status ever since it is conceived. They, however, differ from the conservatives in holding that although the foetus has full moral status, abortion cannot be said to be morally impermissible in all cases. These moderates believe that some cases of abortion may be regarded as permissible on grounds of self-defence.

The second moderate view, which may be regarded as the moderation of the liberal standpoint, upholds that although a foetus does not enjoy significant moral status even in advanced stages of pregnancy, abortion cannot be said to be morally permissible in all cases. These moderates argue that since the foetus is not a person having moral rights, the question of violation of its rights does not arise, but practice of abortion continues to raise moral problems because it has negative social consequences. Late abortions may have harmful effect on those involved and may also erode respect for human life. This moderate view holds that in the early stage of pregnancy a foetus is very much unlike a person, but the same cannot be said about a foetus who may be born within a week or so. According to this moderate view the strongest anti-abortion argument is the one that draws attention to the similarities between a foetus and a baby. The anti-abortionists are on the strongest ground when they urge us to be sympathetic to the fetus. Premature infants and foetus about to be born have so much similarity that it is difficult to draw sharp distinctions between them and offer altogether different treatments to them. Thus, abortion, on this view, is permissible in some cases, while not permissible in some others. Thus it would be wrong to abort a seven months old foetus simply because the mother does not want to postpone a trip to distant country. An early abortion, on the other hand, with the foetus hardly resembling a baby, may be justified if the pregnancy goes against the interests of the mother or of the family. Again, a foetus in the middle period of pregnancy starts resembling a baby, and abortions at this stage can be justified only if continuing the pregnancy would harm the woman physically, psychologically or from a socio-economic point of view. A very late abortion is permissible only if it saves a woman from severe injury or death.

Let us now consider another moderate view which is associated with what is known as 'drawing-the-line' controversy, i.e. the controversy regarding the line that should be drawn between a foetus and a person. We have seen earlier that the conservatives tend to draw the line between a person (a being that has full moral status) and foetus (a being who has no moral status) at conception. The liberals, on the other hand, tend to draw the line either at birth or some time after birth. The third moderate view which we are now considering insists on drawing the line somewhere between the two opposite poles held by the conservatives and the radicals. On this view the line of distinction between a foetus and a person may be drawn at the time when the foetus is implanted on the uterus, or the time when the activity of brain begins, or the time these moderates carry on their speculation regarding the line within a wide range, and their stands accordingly will be different. Those who insist on drawing the line at the time of implantation would uphold a moderate view towards the conservative position, while those who want to draw the line at the time when the foetus becomes viable, would uphold a moderate view with a liberal tinge. The question of moral acceptability of abortion arises when the point where the line of distinction is to be drawn is settled. If abortions are performed before the point is reached, they will be seen as morally acceptable, but abortions that done after the crucial time cannot be said to be morally justified.

We turn now to consider the last of the moderate views discussed in literature on abortion. This moderate view is upheld by those who believe that the foetus has a partial moral status.[6] The proponents of this type of view *reject the 'tissue' theory* which says that the foetus is nothing but *mere pieces of tissue*, having no human significance or value. Zygotes and embryos, they argue, have a *uniqueness distinct from the uniqueness from the body of mother*, they are genetically and organically distinct from the body of the mother, they have the potentiality to develop into person.

This view further, contends that a respect for the sanctity of human life should also discourage us from seeing the foetus as having no moral status. Although the foetus does not qualify as a person, it is nevertheless an 'important and valuable' form of human life and can be said to have a partial moral status.

Of all the views that have been discussed regarding the moral status of the foetus, the last variety of the moderate view seems most plausible and we shall now explain why we are inclined to support this view. We believe that every person would have respect for the sanctity of human life, and although the foetus is not a full-fledged person, it does have a practical moral status. Its significance and value as a form of human life should not be overlooked. At the same time we also believe that every person, as autonomous being, should have the right to make free decisions regarding his or her own life. Every woman has a right to control her own body. She is free to decide when she wants to be a mother and also to decide the number of children she wants to give birth to. We all know that most societies do not take adequate welfare measures for unwanted children. It is somewhat hypocritical on the part of society to condemn abortion and let unwanted children be born in the first place, and then be indifferent and give no importance to their well-being and happiness. Before abortion was legalized many women had to take the help of quacks to get abortion done in a clandestine manner, and most of these abortions were carried out without adequate medical supervision. Recent world health statistics show that about one-fourth to one-third of maternal deaths are caused by complications of abortions that are carried out illegally or without adequate medical competence. Legalization of abortion has considerably lowered the rate of such maternal deaths.

It is true that abortion should not be seen as an easy method of birth control particularly in view of the fact that various contraceptive measures have been developed and made available to people at large. But the point to be noted is that in some cases conception does take place even when birth control measures are followed carefully. According to survey report published by the Indian Council of Medical Research in 1981, 14.5 per cent of women conceive due to contraceptive failure. In such cases abortion becomes the only possible way in which a woman can free herself from an unwanted pregnancy. Decisions regarding abortions should be private decisions.[7] A woman should allow to make her own decision regarding her abortion. The way a woman answers questions about the justifiability of abortion depends considerably on her self-evaluation and her philosophy of life.

Abortion not only involves issues regarding a woman's individual freedom; it also raises social issues. While every woman should have respect for the sanctity of human life, she also has certain duties to herself, her family and her society. If a woman comes to know beforehand that she will give birth to a handicapped child, she is justified in opting for an abortion, not only for her personal happiness, but also for the well-being of society at large. Termination of unwanted pregnancies may also be seen as a duty that one owes to society particularly in view of the fact that population explosion is an acute global problem, and as we have pointed out earlier, the necessity of abortion cannot be questioned on the ground of availability of contraceptive measures because such measures do fail sometimes in spite of being followed carefully.

REFERENCES

1. Jonathan Glover. *Causing Death and Saving Lives,* Penguin. Harmondsworth, 1977, p.122.
2. *Ibid.*, p.125.
3. Peter Singer. *Practical Ethics,* Cambridge University Press Cambridge. 1979, p.109.
4. Glover. *op.cit.*, p.126.
5. M.A.Warren. 'On the Moral and Legal Status of Abortion' in T.A. Mappes and J.S. Zembaty (ed) *Social Ethics* McGraw Hill, New York,1987, p.14.
6. Daniel Callahan. '*Abortion* Decisions: Personal Morality' in *Social Ethics, op.cit.*, p.22.
7. *Ibid.*

Chapter 2

Female Foeticide : An Ethical Issue

M.P. Chaurasia

The first question that we encounter is to define the term Gender. In other words, the problem will take the form of a question, "What is meant by the term Gender?" Certainly, we all have a preconception about what Gender is–femininity and/or masculinity, maleness or femaleness. Sometimes we begin our understanding of gender rooted in the dichotomy of sex, male or female. Gender is most certainly related to sex and is often treated as though it "derives naturally from being either male or female. The categories of sex and gender radically influence our everyday interactions as well as our larger social organization".

In this context, we should distinguish between those two terms "sex" and "gender", as they are not synonymous. Gentile in his thought provoking article has mentioned this difference in the following manner. The term sex is associated with characteristics of an individual that are rooted in biology, i.e., chromosomes and genes that allow for differences in physical appearance and therefore, for the two categories of male and female. In contrast, gender refers to how social and cultural factors shape our reality and our sense of identity as in grammar, things are categorized on the basis of gender. In this way, gender is a social category of shared meanings about characteristics of maleness and femaleness and the behaviours, attitudes and feelings associated with those characteristics. On the basis of sex, population is divided into two groups or categories.

Thus, we have seen that gender is only a part of our identity, we are also known by and know ourselves by other social categories, such as race, social class, ethnic group, religion or age. We need to recognize that these aspects of identity are related to gender. To understand the impact of gender on identity, we must also understand it with regard to other dimensions that are significant in the formation of individual identity. What expectations others dimension that are significant in the formation of individual identity. What expectations others have of us and what treatment we like to receive from others— these are the salient factors, which influence the formation of identity. Most importantly, identity cannot be divided neatly into category membership. So according to Patricia Hill Collins we should not reduce individual identity to any particular social category, as these aspects of identity are the root of social oppression. She further holds that the categorization of individuals into black *versus* white, male *versus* female, poor *versus* rich, promotes false dichotomies that reduce complex identity to superficial characteristics. Such misunderstanding depends on the postulates like Whites rule Blacks, men are deemed superior to woman and reason is seen as being preferable to emotion. On the basis of such assertions some groups are oppressed more than others. If I have an opportunity to ask I would like to ask, " Which has been most oppressive to you, your status as backward persons or your status as woman?" I think, Indian women experience the negative effects of race, class and gender oppression simultaneously. They are the victims of oppression on the ground of class, race and gender. This gender oppression is structured along with three main dimensions such as the institutional, the symbolic and the individual.

Even today such practice has not been stopped and it is a challenge for those who want to change the Indian society. Women may belong to elite family, middle class family or working class family of India suffers equally and such suffering is going on constantly. In 1960s, women in the New Left organization began to extend prior talk about women's rights into the more encompassing discussion of women's liberation, they encountered the fear and hostility of their male comrades and the use of Marxist political theory as support for these reactions. In response to this practical socio-political problem, radical feminists such as Shulamith Firestone invoked biological differences between women and men to explain sexism. She made emphasis on the fact that gender conflict was the most basic form of human conflict and the source of all other forms, including class conflict. She drew not the pervasive tendency within modern culture to locate the roots of gender differences in biology. Her move was to use biologism to establish the primacy of the struggle against male domination rather than to justify tacit concurrence. Later on this move was supported by Anthropologist like Gayle Rubin, who insisted on the fact that we should formulate a theory that could be accounted for the oppression of women in its " endless variety and monotonous similarity." In 1974, an anthropological collection. "Women, Culture and Society" came into the existence which mentioned that women were confined only to the home affairs since the beginning of the civilization and men were provided enough rights to go outside, so, they generated political structures. Rosaldo argued that " while in many societies women possess some or even a great deal of power, women is always viewed as illegitimate, disruptive and without authority."

After 1970s, the movement took a solid shape and it is brought under post-modern thought. The chief advocates of this theory are Michel Foucault, Derrida and Lacan. Basically post-modernism is not a philosophical teaching, rather it is propounded to cut short the status of philosophy. Before 1960, every kind of theory came from philosophy, but onwards every subject has developed theory. Now the definition of theory has been changed, "Theory" means, holds Jonathan Culler", the things either related to psychology, political, or philosophical text or certain names to be considered as authorities like Foucault, Jacques Derrida Lacan. Theory means the view, which is able to explain the problem of other fields except its original field. Works regarded as theory have effects beyond their original field." Now theories are based either on 'sex', 'writing' or 'experience'.

In this way feminism is also a theory, which is based on sex differentiation. The basic postulate, upon which post-modernism depends, is the significant analysis of 'self' and 'other'. Now-a-days, everyone has a deep sense of self, which constituted in early childhood through one's interactions with one's primary parent and which remains relatively constant thereafter. This deep sense of self differs significantly with regard to men and women but is roughly similar among women. This deep sense of self also colours everything one does, as self-awareness signifies one's masculine or feminine gender identity. If masculinity and femininity constitute our basic and every present sense of self, then it is not surprising that the manifestations of sexism are systemic.

Post-modernism as described by Riger is an emerging alternative to rational and empirical analysis. A fundamental assumption of post-modernism is that science 'creates' reality through the imposition of a preconceived view of reality. According to it science should be perceived as the ultimate truth, and its vision often dominates society, especially women and minorities, Post-modernists are more condemned with analyzing power relationship than with uncovering empirical truths, which they claim do not exist. Post-modernism is closely allied with social *constructionism,* sharing the view that gender is multiply constructed. The success of a post-modern analysis is not judged according to the criteria used to judge an empirical analysis. Theory and research can be judged by moral criteria or by the pragmatic utility of the research in achieving a desired outcome. As famous feminist Gergen holds that feminism is a social and political philosophy that advocates challenges to prevailing power dynamic research that allows progress towards these goals would be valued. From a post-modern perspective, it is not meaningful to pose questions about sex differences because the categories of male and female are based on a pre-conceived dualism, the analysis of which serves to reproduce these categories. The study of gender as sex differences also obscures important differences in power among women and among men. Here 'power' implies several meanings. Sometimes it means wealth-power, sometimes knowledge-power and sometimes it means political-power.

Now we shall consider the problem in the above light in Indian perspective, especially in the context of female infanticide. In Indian society 'political power' and 'wealth power' have played a vital role. Michel Foucault has argued that the rise of parliamentary institutions and of new conception of political liberty were accompanied by a darker counter movement, by the emergence of a new unprecedented discipline directed against the body. Everybody has been born either male or female, but not masculine or feminine. Femininity is an artifice or an achievement. Foucault further argued that the transition from traditional to modern societies has been characterized by a profound transformation in the exercise of power, by what he calls "a reversal of the political axis of individuation".

Now in the light of power and individuality we shall consider the condition of Indian femininity. In Indian society there are four *varnas*; Brahmins, Kshatriya, Vaishya and Shudras but I think, our society has also a fifth *varna*, i.e.,*female*. The gents of every *varna* have oppressed them equally. From the very dawn of the Indian civilization we find an apathetic attitude towards our female members. Grammarian like Yaska used the term *duhita/durehita* in a peculiar sense which means daughter must live on a far distance. According to Durgacharya Sahityataraiva *deyate ttravia durhita bhavati* which means, where she goes there she has been upbraided. The term *duhita* signifies the nature of daughter, i.e. always a tendency to borrow something from her father. In some old mythological books, girls are not much respected. In *Aitreya Brahmin*, it is mentioned that, *kripann hi duhita, jyotirhi putrah.* All these references belong to the Brahmin books and old Vaiyakarana period, which is historically regarded as post-Vedic era. Even in *Manusmriti* we find contradictory views regarding women. He restricted the status of women and suggested that a woman should be regarded as a goddess.

So is the case in medieval period. Hatred towards the female of post-Vedic era developed in the form of girl's killing. Such practice came into existence during the Turkish and Persian invasions. It is said that one of the early Muslim invaders of Jharaja's dominated areas, who were experiencing the determination with which they defended their powers, "united policy to arms", and sought to consolidate their vested interest in that particular region by demanding the beautiful daughters of King in marriage. The high-spirited Jadeja aristocrats could not brook the disgrace. And they pretended that they did not preserve their daughters. But they were fearful of the consequences, that force, would be resorted to, listened to their Rajguru in this extremity and put their daughters to death. When the king showed aversion to the murder of a woman, the Rajguru deluded the King by the "fictitious" responsibility, which he accepted and the practice of female infanticide had since then originated. And till the eleventh century and onwards, the repeated Muslim invasions and their rule led to further deterioration in the position of women. Now the killing of girls' child expanded to the entire royal Rajput's family. Orthodox Hindu society was constantly threatened by the fear of the invader's attacks on women. All the elite Hindu family began to hide their daughters behind the curtains. The birth of a daughter was unwelcome because she was considered to be a cause of expense, troubles and anxiety to her parents, since they were merely a custodian till her marriage. Here, we find that the cause of female infanticide was power and wealth.

The Britishers first located female infanticide in India in 1789 in the Varanasi division of the northwestern provinces. Jonathan Ducan found during his official tour of Jaunpur district that the Raj Kumar Rajputs killed their female infants. Subsequently, in early nineteenth century the Britishers found female infanticide to be prevalent among Jadeja Rajputs of Kutch and Kathiawad. By 1850, several castes in north India such as the Jats, Ahirs, Gujars and Khutris, and the Lewapatidar, Kanbis in central Gujarat were found to practice female infanticide.

In the light of above discussed facts, we can understand that female infanticide, in India, has its origin in the history of foreign invasions and their rules in India. Certain ruling and warrior communities who were also ruling communities in maximum number in northwestern provinces of India from where invasions were committed, forced, to practice this inhuman and cruel act in order to protect the honour of their female counterparts and also humiliation arising out of this situation. The lust of foreign invaders and some Muslims rulers for beautiful Hindu girls and women, especially queens and princesses, were increasing day-by-day. The story of Padmavati and several acts of *jauhar* committed in India very well support the facts as analyzed above. All martyrdoms of women were committed under the compulsion of our society to save the power, prestige and wealth.

So far the question regarding the origin of female infanticide in India is concerned, there may be lot of controversial opinions we have. Because every kind of opinion depends on the contention of the individual. But we cannot deny the fact that it has become a real phenomenon for the whole of the country due to many reasons, which have developed over a period of time. Now prevalent alarming situation compels us to think over the problem.

It is significant to note that though female infanticide was outlawed more than a century ago, its detection and prevention are virtually impossible despite reports from across the country which testify to its continued prevalence. Some newborn girls still have poisonous berry juice trickled down their throat, others still choke on a larger than usual '*laddoo* forced into their mouths. As per one report, "They (villagers) let the baby starve, or make it lie on the stomach as soon as she is born or to cover the face with wet towel. But more sinister, and perhaps more widespread than the murder of a baby girl is the newest form of violence against her killing even before she is born. Amniocentesis, originally intended as pre-natal test to detect certain genital abnormalities, is now widely used across the country to determine the sex of foetus and abort it if it happens to be a female. In a study of 8,000 abortions after amniocentesis in Bombay it was reported that 799 of the aborted foetuses were female. It is also estimated that 1.20 crore girls are born in India every year. About one-fourth of them die before their fifteenth birthday because of female infanticide, malnutrition, and discrimination in health care and material mortality and as victim of rape and molestation.

Now such practice has reached middle class urban families especially in metropolitan and district towns in India. Perhaps this is the latest form of violence against girl child. Many reports of this sense have been highlighted in several newspapers by different non-government organizations. There are several clinics in every town, which is running in the name of maternity care centres for family health centres. Many reports of this fact were published in a national daily that in 1991 approximately one thousand foetuses were destroyed in India of which nearly 995 were female foetuses. The people, who were indulged in this misdeed, belonged mostly to the educated and well to do family. According to Dr. Sanjeeva Kulkarni of the Foundation Research in Community Health 5,000 amniocentesis tests are carried out in Bombay annually to detect the foetus. Mostly pregnancies were aborted after sex determination of the foetuses in which the number of the female was greater than that of the male. In *India Today*, a report of Anna M.S. Veticad and Ramesh Vinayak was published last year under the title "*Maada Bhrun Hatya Ka Jaari Hai Dhandha*". The report says that more than lac of female foetuses are killed every year in Punjab, Haryana, Chandigarh, U.P. and Uttranchal.

This situation has further taken alarming proportions after the new researches that provide possibility of pre-conception sex-selection technologies. Cashing in on son-preference, a value that is entrenched in Indian society, this new sex-selection procedure has entered the market and 'Gender Selection' is now a reality. As a result of the new techniques the genetic determination has taken an ugly turn. It blocks the path of coming of a female child on the earth in a most sophisticated manner. Several reports reveal this aspect. The status of the girl child is reflected in the juvenile sex ratio, which has registered a sharp decline over the last decade from 945 females per 1000 male in 1991 Census to 927/1000 and now in certain parts of India this ratio is 703:1000 in 2001. Arvind

Jain has mentioned in his report in *Hindustan* "*Kaun sunta hai stri ki cheekh*" presented a horrible fact about female foeticides. In India every year 40,000 new girls, due to poverty, are coming in the job of prostitution.

Many arguments can be forwarded either in favour of such act or against it. Jill and Scott Sweazy, the promoters of a U.S. based 'Gen-Select' company which provides ' Gen-Select Kit' to have a child of desired sex by parents with the help of preconception sex-selection technology has argued that the question of genetic determination is related only to the parents of an incoming child, because it is the liberty of the parents to choose the desired child. She further argued that, "with our product, the freedom to choose the gender of your next child is preserved, while the moral, ethical and legal issues of *foeticide* are put to case." In the same way, various arguments have been advanced by many intellectuals on the basis of utilitarian philosophy. According to this theory human beings are supposed to be guided only by pleasure-pain principle and the only criterion of determination of what is good or bad is the amount of pleasure or pain it gives. So, if the arrival of a male child proves a source of pleasure, the parents should have the freedom to enjoy it. But in Indian context such is not the case. Here the freedom of mother is overpowered by father's desire. Here, utilitarian principle of ethics has not been enjoyed in its true spirit. Parents ignored the freedom of the incoming child. We cannot ask for freedom outside the state and society. So only socially sanctioned freedom must be entertained. Recently the Human Rights Commission has declared the right of life. And this right is ignored in case of a girl child, if she is not allowed to see the world either by abortion of female *Foeticide* or by not allowing her to take shape with the help of pre-conception sex-selection techniques. Several ethical objections have been raised when the misuse of some techniques has already taken place. Ultra-sound is one of those techniques through which such act is performed and this event has taken a form of 'menace' in India. Moral philosopher J.S.Mill also holds that liberty does not mean the liberty of will, it has to work within the framework of society and state. The liberty of the individual must thus far be limited; he must not make himself a nuisance to other people. From my point of view no freedom is possible in the absence of authority and the authority is state, which must be legitimate and not be absolute. I don't want to raise the pros and cons sides of abortions but I want to attract the attention of learned people towards those abortions, which are based on sex-determination. Such abortion is committed only when the incoming child is girl. So, it is an ethical issue. You cannot discriminate a people on the basis of caste, sex and race, as it is related to biology, it is a gift of nature.

In India, the government has exercised a few laws. The Sansad of India has legislated certain laws to stop this misdeed in which some are under consideration. Recently, apex Court of India has passed a judgement against the pre-natal sex-determination test. In it, the Court has decided to impose seven years rigorous imprisonment. In previous panchayats and District Board election certain electoral constituencies were reserved for women and they have been elected too. But so far the exercising of power is concerned, they all have authorized their male relative to enjoy the power. Just I remember Hillary Clinton's address in the beginning on the eve of Fourth World Conference on Women sponsored by U.N.O. In the Indian context she told, " It is a violation of human rights when individual women are doused with gasoline, set on fire and burnt to death because their marriage dowries are deemed to be small, it is a violation of human rights when babies are killed because they are girls, when women are sold into prostitution or raped as prizes in war or subjected to violation in their houses". She further said, "If there is one message that echoes from this conference, let it be that human rights are women's rights and women's rights are human rights once and for all".[29]

We have already discussed all the mishappenings with Indian women from pregnancy to marriage and also some legal remedies related to it. We have also seen that political and legal advantages are unable to stop such injustice. There are certain States in India of which Chief Ministers are women, but even then such heinous crime is going on. If you open the daily newspapers of Bihar, you will find that in Saran range 80 per cent abortion cases are happening due to pre-natal sex-determination test and brides are burnt to death even for a buffalo or a motorcycle. But it is good for the sake of women that a few women of our society have dared to knock the door of the court. But it is not enough.

For the sake of remedy, only the state and courts interventions are not sufficient. There must be some proper ethical consciousness. The women should be empowered with certain rights only that right can stop these activities successfully. The right of maternity and the right of marriage should be wholly granted to women. But to provide with rights is not the proper treatment of this evil. We should also create an ethical environment in which all those reformations may flourish.

So far the ethical consideration is concerned professional philosophy and ethics have equally ignored this problem. Moral philosopher like Kant has separated them by saying 'fair-sex'. But Kant in his theory of knowledge has emphasized the cases of this separation. According to him, knowledge is actively constructed rather than passively received. Time, space, self and other, as well as the categories of developmental theory, all arise out of the active interchange between the individual and the physical and social world in which we live and of which we strive to make sense. The moral judgement is a statement of priority, an attempt at rational resolution in a situation where, from a different point of view, the choice itself seems to do violence to justice. For the sake of moral evolution two conditions are necessary: an individual and his relationship with others. Only a true individual can judge the action properly. The other condition is the capacity to take responsibility as an individual. Actually what Kant meant to say is the above fact? Only taking of one's responsibility and obligation makes his action right or wrong. For the sake of one's personality development, the capacity of mature judging is necessary. But Indian feminine still are passively waiting to happen the event with herself rather than to make the events actively according to her choice. The essence of the moral decision is the exercise of choice and the willingness to accept responsibility for that choice. In this course women have no choices and they correspondingly excuse themselves from the responsibility that decision implied. The conflict between self and other thus constitutes the central moral problem for women, which can only be resolved by reconciliation between femininity and adulthood. Indian women are always ready to take obligations of others like wives and mothers but never as an individual themselves though from the moral point of view only individual's decisions are relevant. Self-realization is the first step of morality and the second level is known as responsibility and obligation. Women should prefer existing by themselves and become self-dependent. In this course the transition from selfishness to responsibility is a move towards social participation. The moralities of men are based on rights till dates while the morality of women are based on duty in India, i.e., duty of sacrifice and nothing else.

Terms like power, control, distribution and their forms have a significant place in modern moral philosophy. In the same way Carol Gilligan emphasizes that power and attachment are two ways of defining relationship, two ways of defining responsibilities. Morality is a perception, it is a thing to follow, and the idea of having a concept of morality is to try to figure out what it is that people can do in order to make life worth living and make for a kind of balance, a kind of equilibrium, a harmony in which everybody feels he has a place and an equal share in things and its doing. It is woman and only woman that bear the responsibility of other Individual's coming in the world. If she herself is ready to take her own responsibility and also of other individuals she does not need the approval of any man at all. Most often, she is harassed and exploited everywhere, not for herself, but for others.

Now-a-days, the updated people have changed the meanings of the terms 'right' and 'wrong'. 'Right' is rooted in law, the world of rights. Good in the relevant sense suggests commerce, the world of goods. So, every kind of ethical theory depends on a special kind of ethical theory, depends on a special kind of relationship that is responsible to the situations. The term friendship is vague one. Sometimes it implies the meaning of sexual intimacy, kinship and a variety of networks loosely dubbed and sometimes personal relationship and informal practices. Indian women need theories of ethics of informal and personal relationships. The informal and the personal relations are the same. An informal agreement need not be personal. An interpersonal relationship is personal when it matters to the either parties and its importance depends on the nature of the relationship. "Personal" suggests closeness and intimacy. A relation is formal to the extent that it is well defined, limited, in a way that are publicly understood and publicly sanctioned. Formality is not the same as legality. Public life relationships are formal while official relationships are informal. So women should take the responsibility as per the importance of the relationship but they must be always aware of their own status. Every path is open, but no other people can lead them to their goal. Only women have to cross the road and attain the goal. Recently, in a personal talk, Dr. M.N.Sinha has told me that in Haryana, society has provided the right of marriage to the girls and there mostly cases of dowry practices have come to a halt.

Chapter 3

Trust and Responsibility in Sexual Ethics in the Context of HIV/AIDS

Devarakonda Balaganapathi

Sexual ethics is an important area of discussion in the contemporary ethical debates. The discussions on sexual ethics gained relevance especially in the context of the rise of Global epidemic of HIV/AIDS, which is threatening the human life at large. Trust and Responsibility form the basic pillars of any human relationship including the relation of sexual partners. This chapter discusses the place of 'trust' and 'responsibility' in the sexual ethics in the context of HIV/AIDS. It argues that only in a single partner, known and long-term relationship trust and responsibility are strong and hence only by adopting such a relationship, it is possible to avoid transmission of AIDS.

Since its early beginning during 1980s in a few places, the human immuno-deficiency virus (HIV) has spread to every continent on earth. As per the report of joint UN program on HIV/AIDS and the World Health Organization, by the beginning of 1998 over 30 million people were infected with HIV, and that 11.7 million people around the world already lost their lives to the disease. The report also mentions that the virus continues to spread, causing nearly 16,000 new infections a day. It further adds that, today one in every 100 adults in the most sexually active age group (15-49) is living with HIV. These facts along with the lack of availability of the cure for the epidemic till now prove the lethality of the disease. This lethality of the epidemic raised the concern of the researchers related to both scientific and non-scientific areas. Finding a cure or preventive medicine has become the concern of scientific research, whereas looking at the ethical aspects, public policy, etc., have become the concern of non-scientific areas of research. This chapter concerns with the ethical issues related to AIDS.

Given that there is no available cure for AIDS and that prevention is the only way to restrict the spread of the disease, there are a number of ethical dilemmas that went on into discussion related to professional ethics as to "What kind of treatment should be given to the HIV infected person"? and "Whether confidentiality has to be maintained regarding the position of the infected person"? etc., which are very much relevant to the medical research. However, along with these issues, a pertinent issue that needs to be discussed, in the context of prevention being the only way to restrict HIV, is sexual ethics. What kind of ethics has to be practiced by the sexual partners? What is the place of trust among the sexual partners? What kind of responsibility sexual partners should have towards each other? etc., are some of the important questions that need to be raised afresh in the context of HIV.

Trust and Responsibility

Trust and responsibility form the basic foundations on which any human relationship is built. Breach of either trust or responsibility would cause ethical concern.

Humans are generally understood to be social beings, which implies that they are involved in multiple relationships. All the codes of conduct whether it be social, religious, moral or institutional, presume some kind of trust between the people involved. In other words, people trust each other involved in a relationship, whether it be friendship or a family relation or some other association, thus, making trust the foundation of every relationship. Trust makes the relationships simpler and the world less dangerous. This has been rightly pointed out by Luhmann (1973) when he noted that, trust lets us inhabit a simpler and less threatening world, a world in which we need not plan for every contingency.

Gambetta (1998:217) while explaining trust in terms of a cooperative action, states that trust is a certain level of subjective probability with which an agent assesses another agent or group of agents who perform a particular action irrespective of his monitoring. It follows that in trust, one has the confident expectation that the other would respond favourably. This seems to be bringing out trust in the context of hierarchical conditions. Trust proceeds from the belief that the person on whom trust is reposited would behave as per the expectations. For instance, when X trusts Y, X believes that Y will behave in a certain expected way. In other words, Y is expected by X to behave in a certain way. This assumes that there is some kind of relationship between X and Y, and Y is trusted by X on the belief that Y would behave in a certain way. What is to be noted in this relationship is that, if X trusts Y, it doesn't consequently follow that Y also has to trust X. Instead, Y gets into an obligation to keep the trust of Y. This obligation is justified only when Y knows about the trust that Y reposited. So mutual knowledge and mutual understanding qualifies this obligation.

Given that trust requires a kind of mutual knowledge and understanding, if the relation from X to Y is trust, then what is the relation from Y to X. This brings us to another important notion of obligation called 'responsibility'. Knowledge of X's trust would make Y to be responsible; to be responsible to keep the trust and live up to the expectations of X. In other words, if X trusts Y, then Y is bound by the responsibility towards X. To be responsible for something is to be answerable for it. A responsible person is someone who can be trusted to discharge their prospective responsibilities, and to accept their retrospective responsibilities. Prospective responsibilities are the things which are up to us to attend to and are attached to particular roles (as parents or doctors) or responsibilities we have as moral agents. Retrospective responsibilities are attributed to things that we have done or failed to do. Prospective responsibilities are applied to future course of actions and retrospective responsibilities are attributed to past deeds. Trust can only be reposited with regard to prospective responsibilities. There are two preconditions to make a person responsible to a person who trusted him; they are, on the one hand the knowledge of the trust that is reposited and on the other hand things should be under agents control to act.

Following the above discussion, it can be understood that whenever there is trust there ought to be responsibility and wherever there is responsibility trust would definitely exist there. Trust and responsibility are, thus, the two sides of any relationship. Breach of any of these two would lead to the collapse of the relationship. Mistrust and irresponsibility would make the life of a person miserable by destroying all social relations.

As there are a number of relationships into which a person can enter in any particular given time, it would be interesting to understand whether trust and responsibility remain same with regard to all relationships. All human relationships can possibly be divided into two kinds; relationships with known people and relationships with unknown people. X is said to be in a known relationship with Y if both X and Y know each other. X is said to be in an unknown relationship with Y if either or both of them do not know the other. Relationship between known people can be subdivided into family relations and outside family relations such as friends, relations, etc. In the relationship between unknown people either one of them may know the other indirectly, or both of them may not know each other.

Trust and responsibility are very strong in known relationships and they seem to be frail in unknown relationships. Even among the known relationships, family relations are the strongest and outside family relations are comparatively less strong. Let us stop our discussion on the role of trust and responsibility in a relationship in general and let us concentrate on a particular relationship which is one of the most basic and is supposed to be an essential form of all relationships that is sexual relationship.

The philosophy of sex begins with a picture of a privileged pattern of relationship in which two adults love each other and are faithful to each other. X and Y are said to be sexually related only when both are involved in a sexual act. Intimacy and privacy being the core features, sexual relationship brings together the sexual partners and puts them under obligation to one another. Intimacy involved in this relationship requires privacy and privacy and intimacy make this relationship different from and unique among the other relationships. As it is the case with any other relationship sexual partners also have trust and responsibility towards each other. However, unlike other kinds of relations, sexual relations, since they are qualified by intimacy and privacy, are mutual. That is, to say that, X and Y are involved in a sexual relation implies that X trusts Y and that Y has responsibility of keeping the trust of X. Furthermore, it also implies that Y also trusts X and X also has responsibility of keeping the trust of Y. What follows from this analysis is that both the sexual partners ought to have trust and responsibility towards the other. This makes the sexual relationship stronger than any other relationship.

Appearance of AIDS on the global scene has set the need for looking at sexual ethics afresh as its transmission is also through the sexual relationship. The need arose because, as it is noted, "AIDS is no 'ordinary' epidemic. More than a devastating disease, it is freighted with profound social and cultural meaning. More than a passing tragedy, it will have long term, broad-ranging effects on personal relationships, social institutions, and cultural configurations". The above note explicates the lethality of the epidemic and indirectly points to the loss of trust and responsibility which may have long-term effects on personal relationships, social institutions and cultural configurations. Due to this lethality there is a subtle shift in the sexual ethics that has occurred in the recent times. Ronald Bayer (1999) while noting this shift stated that, in the early years of the epidemic people were reluctant to discuss the moral responsibility of HIV infected people to warn or to protect their sexual partners. Instead, the accent was on the more egoistic goal of self-protection. Part of the rationale for this approach was a concern that HIV infected people, already subject to stigmatization, would have unique duties imposed on them by an intolerant society. Bayer applauds the recent development of a more balanced, mature and altruistic ethic that includes attention to the welfare of others. However, he notes that ambiguities remain, especially regarding the role of trust in sexual ethics. Though it is true that, thanks to the efforts of international organizations such as UN and WHO and the respective states in bringing awareness, there is a subtle shift in the sexual ethics from egoistic self-preservation to a mature, balanced and altruistic ethics, what needed to be stressed is the role of trust and responsibility in sexual ethics. Along with the discussion on the responsibilities of HIV infected people, a healthy relationship between the sexual partners with complete trust and responsibility ought to be stressed. Given the discussion on trust and responsibility above let us understand what kind of relationship ought to be adopted by the sexual partners to prevent the spread of AIDS.

Since sexual relationship is an intimate and private one, the partners are equally obliged to each other. Both are not only responsible for the act, but are also equally responsible for the consequences. To be responsible to the other and to be trusted by the other one ought to restrict the number of sexual partners to one. Involving in sexual relation with more than one partner would lead to the betrayal of trust and responsibility.

Trust and responsibility are stronger, as it is discussed above, in a known relationship, especially in a family relationship. In a relationship between known people parties involved would have the knowledge of trust and responsibility towards each other. In a sexual relationship more than mere knowledge of trust and responsibility involvement in facing the consequences is needed. This involvement is available only in a married family relationship. In a marriage relationship, the partners have to trust each other, know their responsibilities and face the consequences of their actions. Since the family relationship is a closed one involving only the partners the consequences would directly and readily fall on them, putting them under serious obligation.

Further, trust and responsibility would be strong only in a long-term relationship. In a short-term relationship, since the partners would know that they may not continue in the relationship for long, there is a chance for betrayal. It may many times end before the consequences come up. Only in a long-term relationship, since both partners have to face the consequences together, there would be mutual trust and mutual feeling of responsibility.

Conclusion

To sum up, appearance of AIDS epidemic has necessitated the need to look at the sexual ethics afresh. Given the lethality of the disease and lack of cure, and prevention being the only way to stop, a good and healthy sexual relationship could only save the sexual partners from this epidemic. It is argued that intimacy and privacy which are the core features of sexual relationship puts the sexual partners under obligation to one another. Trust and responsibility which are the basic foundations of any relationship especially sexual relationship, necessitates one partner, known and long-term relationship in order to avoid the spread of AIDS.

NOTES

1. LeRoy Walters. 1999. "Ethical Issues in the Prevention and Treatment of HIV Infection and AIDS" in *Contemporary Issues in Bioethics* (V end) eds. Tom L Beauchamp and LeRoy Walters, Belmont; Wadsworth Publishing Company.
2. Ronald Bayer and Jeff Stryker. 1999. "Ethical Challenges posed by Clinical Progress in AIDS" in *Contemporary Issues in Bioethics* (V end) eds. Tom L Beauchamp and LeRoy Walters, Belmont; Wadsworth Publishing Company.
3. Susan and Cochran and Vickie M. Mays. 1999. "Sex, Lies and HIV". in *Contemporary Issues in Bioethics* (V end) eds. Tom L Beauchamp and LeRoy Walters, Belmont; Wadsworth Publishing Company.
4. Ronald Bayer, 1999. "AIDS Prevention – Sexual Ethics and Responsibility" in *Contemporary Issues in Bioethics* (V end) eds. Tom L Beauchamp and LeRoy Walters, Belmont; Wadsworth Publishing Company.

5. Tom L Beauchmp & LeRoy Walters 1999. (eds) *Contemporary Issues in Bioethics* (V end) Belmont; Wadsworth Publishing Company.
6. Ferdinand Schocman. 1999. "AIDS and Privacy" in *Contemporary Issues in Bioethics* (V end) eds. Tom L Beauchamp and LeRoy Walters, Belmont; Wadsworth Publishing Company.
7. Mackinnon, Barbara 2001. *Ethics: Theory and Contemporary Issues*. Belmont: Wadsworth/Thomson Learning.
8. Harris, J & Holm S. 1995. "Is there a moral obligation not to infect others?" *BMJ*. 311 (7014). 1215-1217.
9. Stein, M.D., Freadberg KA, Sullivan L.M, Savetsky J, Levenson S.M., Hingson R. & Samet J.H. 1995. "Sexual Ethics: Disclosure of HIV-Positive Status to Partners" *Archives of Internal Medicine*. 158 (3). 253-7.
10. Luhmann, N. 1973. "Trust: A Mechanism for the Reduction of Social Complexity", Trans H Davis, J Raffman, K Rooney, T. Burns & G. Poggi eds. *Trust and Power*. Chichester, NY: Wiley.
11. Gambetta, 1998. "Can We Trust Trust?" in D Gambetta (ed) *Trust: Making and Breaking Cooperative Relations*. New York: Blackwell.
12. Russell, Bertrand. 1965. *Marriage and Morals*. London: Unwin Books.
13. Dorothy Nelkin, David P Willis & Scott V. Parris. 1999. "Introduction" in Dorothy Nelkin, David P Willis & Scott V. Parris (eds.) *A Disease of Society: Cultural and Institutional Responses to AIDS*. New York: Cambridge University Press.

Chapter 4

Euthanasia: An Ethical Issue

Pratima Ganguli

It is a universal truth that where there is life, there is death. If a living thing is born, it must die in the long run. Death is a part of life. It is an uncompromising condition for everybody born on earth. Among many causes of death, disease is an important one. Although due to the advancement of medical science many new techniques are invented and powerful medicines are available in the market. Thus doctors have succeeded largely in curing so many serious types of diseases. But still, death is inevitable. Man is mortal. Very often death comes in such a cruel way that the affected person has to undergo in terrible pain or to remain in 'coma' for a long period. In such circumstances, even the doctors are unable to save the person's life. They are helpless in this situation. Here comes the question of euthanasia. The patient wishes to die rather than to live in a painful condition. A handicapped life is nothing but a burden on the patient, parents and society, so the patient may willingly opt for death. In case of an infant, euthanasia takes place with the consent of parents also.

The word 'euthanasia' comes from Greek, which means 'easy death', 'gentle death' or 'happy death'. As per dictionary meaning, it does not refer to only a normal death of a man in his old age but to the killing of a man whether it is an infant or a grown up man who is suffering from such pain and disease, which is incurable. The term 'euthanasia' has come to be applied specifically in the medical field to the intentional killing of a human being for the purpose of ending his/her suffering or of removing some burden. Peter Singer in his book writes about euthanasia "It is now used to refer to the killing of those who are incurably ill and a great pain or disease, for the sake of those killed, and in order to spare them further suffering of distress".

Dr. Richard Lamerton, former Director of St. Joseph's Hospice Home Care Service in London has stated that in using the term euthanasia to stand for both 'mercy killing' and allowing someone 'to die', we seriously raise a very necessary and important distinction between an act of murder and what is merely good medical practice (allowing people to die of natural causes, without using any extraordinary or heroic measures to keep them alive)".

Thus, 'euthanasia' is a confusing and ambiguous term, because it is subject to emotionalism. So, in *Ethics: Theory and Practice* Jacques Thiroux has substituted three other phrases: 'Allowing someone to die', 'Mercy death' and 'Mercy killing'. 'Allowing someone to die' implies an essential recognition that there is some point in any terminal illness when further curative treatment has no purpose and that a patient in this situation should be allowed to die a natural death in comfort, peace and dignity. It means, allowing a terminally ill patient to die his or her own natural death without interference from medical science and technology. 'Mercy death' is the taking of a direct action in order to terminate a patient's life because the patient has requested it. It is really an assisted suicide. And 'mercy killing' is the taking of a direct action to terminate a patient's life without his or her permission. This type of action is often made on the assumption that the patient's life is no longer 'meaningful'.

As we know that euthanasia is neither suicide nor murder. Although sometimes it is termed as *assisted suicide* as the affected person needs help from others to end his or her life. When a person suffers from incurable disease and longs for death hopelessly, the euthanasia in such circumstances is only a way out. Generally suicide is believed to be a cowardice act, which is performed without least considering other persons who are dependent on him or her. And Murder is totally different from suicide. It is forced on someone against his or her wishes. The victim ordinarily remains ignorant about the impending danger of death. Generally the murder is committed out of vengeance or for some templation. It is certainly a social evil.

Thus, euthanasia is neither suicide nor murder but it is denoted by 'mercy killing' or 'mercy death'. Although Jacques Thiroux has made a distinction between these two by saying "the important distinction between mercy killing and 'mercy death' is that 'mercy killing' is involuntary or does not involve the patient's permission or request, whereas 'mercy death' is done with the permission of the patient, and usually at his or her request".

On the basis of above discussion, euthanasia may be categorised as different types. These are voluntary, involuntary and non-voluntary euthanasia.

(i) Voluntary Euthanasia

As per voluntary euthanasia death is carried out at the request of the person concerned. The patient agreed to be killed or requested for it. If there is such a request or agreement the euthanasia is called voluntary. For example, Jean, wife of Humphry was dying of cancer and not able to bear severe pain. She asked her husband to end her life who obtained some tablets and gave them to Jean, she took the tablets and died soon afterwards. Sometimes people want to die, but unable to kill themselves. An incident occurred in New Jersey in the year 1973. George was injured in a motor cycle accident. He was taken to hospital and was found to be totally paralysed from the neckdown. He was also in severe pain and told his doctor that he did not want to live in this condition. His brother blessed him, then smuggled a gun into the hospital and shot him. Dr. Jack Kevorkian, Michigan pathologist went one step further when he built a suicide machine to help terminally ill people to end their lives. This was a case of assisted suicide, which was not against the law of Michigan. But before accepting death the terminally ill people had to express his/her wish to end life. Although there should be some procedure of voluntary euthanasia purpose. But sometimes without that also it happens as in case of George in above examples.

Euthanasia can be voluntary even if a person is not able, as in case of Jean and George, to indicate the wish to die right up the moment the tablets swallowed or the trigger pulled. A person may, while in good health make a written request for euthanasia, if through accident or illness he/she becomes incapable of making or expressing a decision to die. In killing such a person one could truely to be acting with the consent of the person concerned.

(ii) Involuntary Euthanasia

When the person killed is capable of consenting to his or her own death, but does not do so either because not asked or because the person expressed another desire is known as involuntary euthanasia. It is involuntary where the person killed refuses or otherwise actively withholds consent (again, whether this be at the time of the killing or in an advance directive), or where person could have asked whether he consented, but was not asked. In any case we should be very particular about the motive for killing, which of course should be the desire to prevent unbearable suffering on the part of the person killed. Although genuine cases of involuntary euthanasia appear to be very rare.

(iii) Non-voluntary Euthanasia

The above two forms of euthanasia leave room for a third kind of the same when a person is not capable of understanding the choice between life and death, euthanasia would be neither voluntary nor involuntary, but non-voluntary. This happens in the case of the people who due to some reasons have permanently lost the capacity to understand the issue involved, without having previously requested or rejected euthanasia in these circumstances. Several cases of non-voluntary euthanasia have reached the courts and in the press in many countries. Louis had a son who was described as 'incurable imbecile' and had been ridden since infancy and 'blind for five years.' According to Louis his son was like dead all the time, could not talk, could not walk. At last he himself killed his son by giving him chloroform.

An infant named Samuel was admitted to a hospital in Chicago, in the year 1986, who swallowed a small object that struck in his wind pipe cousing loss of oxygen to his brain. He was completely in a camatose for eight months and placed on a respirator. One day his parents visited the hospital and soon after his mother left the room, the father while cradling the baby in his arms disconnected him from the respirator till death. Here we observe that there is no desire to die on the part of the infant concerned. So the question naturally arises whether the euthanasia here is for the baby or for the sake of the family? In both the cases the brains were so damaged that the lives of the babies were incapable of recovery. Hence, it is for the well-being of their families that the babies are allowed to die.

After a brief discussion on the term 'Euthanasia' and its different forms let us now try to focus on the moral questions involved in its. We know that the question of Euthanasia form an important part of biomedical ethics which again is a sub-part of Applied Ethics, very much discussed in present century.

The pertinent moral question which can be raised here is that whether Euthanasia is morally justified or not? While giving answer to the above question the moral philosophers are divided broadly in *two groups*, namely *liberal and conservative*. Before discussing the view points of both the groups one should be very particular regarding the basic moral question in this matter, i.e., consent of person concerned. In any case whether it is voluntary, Involuntary or non-voluntary, euthanasia, first of all we should be very prompt and particular about the opinion of concerned persons who are directly involved in it. Now, we must discuss the view-points of the liberal groups who support euthanasia and give the following arguments in its favour.

(i) Individual Freedom and Rights

They say that it is right and freedom of individual to take decision whether they will live or die. If they think it is better to die than to live and request other to kill then it does not fall under the section of crime. If we kill them at their request it will be based on love, compassion or mercy. J. Thirroux has quoted a view of a doctor which is remarkable here—"I remember hearing a doctor expressing this point of view on a television documentary called Right to Die. The doctor said, "you have the right to choose death for yourself, but you do not have the right to involve me in your choice."

(ii) Mercy for the 'living dead'

This argument for mercy killing states that the man who is going to be killed is not fully alive. He is half-dead and devoid of all strength, movement and mental expression. The mercy killing may be related to the cases as brain damage, paralysis of whole body, complete kidney failure, etc. Even if such people recover from their comas, the damage to their brains is so extensive that their lives will never again be normal. They will have a plantlike existence, exhibiting no personality or real human consciousness. Whatsoever; therefore, it is an act of mercy to end their existence.

(iii) Financial and Emotional Burdens

The medical care and treatment of greater and incurable diseases is too expensive and naturally it is financial and emotional burden upon the concerned family and society. Such burden is so heavy sometimes that a well-to-do family becomes pauper and cannot progress in other lives or fields.

(iv) Human Rights versus Animal Rights

Another argument states that just as we are generally willing to put animals out of their misery when they suffer, so we should accord our fellow humans, the same consideration. Furthermore, because they have asked us for death, we should have no compunction about ending their lives mercifully.

(v) The Right to Die with Dignity

Another argument for allowing someone to die is that people have the right to die with dignity rather than waste away and suffer until there is little left of their original character. This argument is especially forceful in relation to long-term debilitating and degenerative diseases, such as cancer. The argument states further that 'dignity' also is achieved when patients are given choices concerning the kind of living, dying they will do.

It is a common notion that human life is always to be safeguarded and preserved. Persons who think so are against allowing someone to die. Their arguments are as follows:

(i) Abandonment of Patients

If the health care professionals such as doctors, do not apply curative treatments, they are responsible for abandoning patients to suffer miseries. They are of opinion that allowing someone to die means refusal of proper medical care. Doctors should continue medical treatment as long as there is life in the patient.

(ii) The Possibility of Finding Cures

J. Thiroux argues that if we are too quick to let people die, we may be denying them the opportunity to be cured of their illness. New cures for disease are constantly being discovered, and there are also so called 'miracle cures', that is, cures that occur in seeming defiance of all medical knowledge. Therefore, we continue every effort to keep dying patients alive, a miracle cure may occur, or a scientific cure (new drug or surgical procedure) may be discovered that will lengthen patients lives or even cure them completely.

(iii) The Impossibility of Opting for Death

Many persons think that it is wrong to exercise option for death, rather we should always select life. In their views the function of medicines is to save life, not to bring the life to death. The purpose of medicine is nullified as soon as we start to make the choice for death. It creates discouragement in doctors in one hand and arouse distrust of patient in doctors on the other hand.

(iv) Interference with God's Divine Plan

Another argument against allowing somebody to die lies in the fact that life and death are caused by God and a man cannot take away one's life which is given by God only, we must use all our abilities and best methods to protect, preserve and prolong man's life until God precipitates the patient's death.

(v) The Irrationality of Mercy Death

The patient suffering from any disease of pain and misery should not be disappointed so soon and should not take decision to be dead so early. Generally such people who decide to die are in a state of fear and depression and they are not able to think in a proper way. They lack rational decision.

(vi) Direct Violation of the Value of Life Principle

Mercy killing is a direct violation of the value of life principle, especially because, unlike defense of the innocent, war, and capital punishment, it usually involves taking the life of an innocent person. As in the mercy death situation, the argument here is that murder is murder regardless of motive, therefore, mercy killing is nothing less than pre-meditated murder.

Now, a question may be raised regarding the justification of euthanasia. Different thinkers are of different opinion in this matter. According to some, euthanasia may be allowed as it gives relief to the persons who are incurably ill, if in their cases medical science is totally helpless. As we have earlier said that the competence of doctor cannot be final and his decision and diagnosis cannot be accepted ultimately and eventually. A doctor may fail in finding out the root cause or kind of disease or in treatment. His knowledge about medical science or the process of healing may be imperfect in some particular case. In this situation the justification of euthanasia may be doubtful.

There are thinkers who are strictly against euthanasia. They say that no human being has any right to end his own life, as life is precious gift of God. For any direct or indirect interest man should not treat himself as an end as Kant has said. John Louder in this regard says, "I wholly disagree with euthanasia. Though it is fully logical, and in expert and conscientious hands it could be the most humane way of dealing with such a situation. But legalizing euthanasia would be a most dangerous weapon in the hands of the state or ignorant or unscrupulous individuals. One does not have to go far back in history to know what crimes can be committed if euthanasia were legalised". According to Peter Singer, there is a conflict between the two views as given below:

(i) To protect the sanctity of human life.
(ii) To aim at reducing suffering and pain.

If we accept the first point the second is neglected and if the second point is accepted the first is ignored. If naturally a man is born and dies there is no complain against it. Immatured but natural death is out of the control of euthanasia which does not come under blame and criticism. We believe in the fact that life and death are in the hands of God. Natural or normal death cannot create any controversy or cannot divide critics into two groups as in the case of euthanasia. Here the moralists disagree, religious viewpoints vary and medical practice is inconsistent: Even in legal matters, law as it is written and law as it is practiced are vastly different. According to Rath and Russell the best solution is to exact comprehensive euthanasia law, one that would provide for active and passive euthanasia and that would meet a broad-spectrum of needs.

Hence, if mercy death is to be allowed, there should be a guarantee that it would be morally and legally permissible.

NOTES

Baruch Brody, ed., *Suicide and Euthanasia*, Norwel, MA: Kluwer Academic Publications, 1989.

David S. Oderbery, *Applied Ethics: A Non-Consequentialist Approach*; Blackwell, USA, 2000.

George H. Kieffer, Bioethics: *A Textbook of Issues*; Addison-Wesley Publishing Company, London, 1979.

Jacques Thirous, Ethics: *Theory and Practice*, Prentice Hall, 1998.

John A. Behnke and Sissela Bok, *The Dilemmas of Euthanasia*; Garden City, NY: Anchor Books, 1975.

John H. Piet and Ayodhya Prasad, *Introduction to Applied Ethics*, Cosmo Publications, India, 2000.

James Rachels, *The End of Life: Euthanasia and Morality*, Oxford University Press, New York, 1986.

Peter Byrne, *Philosophical and Ethical Problems in Mental Handicap*, Macmillan Press Ltd., 2000.

Peter Singer, Practical Ethics, Cambridge University Press, 1993.

Peter Singer, (ed.), *A Companion to Ethics*, Blackwell Oxford, 2000.

Journal, *Pariksha Manthan and Ichchha Mrityu*, Venkatesh Prakasan', 2005.

Chapter 5

Euthanasia : A Moral Analysis

Shiva Bhanu Singh

The term euthanasia comes from the Greek words '*eu*' and '*thanatos*' which combined means, "Good death", or a gentle and easy death. Hippocrates mentions euthanasia in the *Hippocratic Oath*, which was written between 400 and 300 B.C. The original Oath states : "To please no one will I prescribe a deadly drug nor give advice which may cause his death". Euthanasia is a practice of terminating the life of a person in a painless or minimally painful way in order to stop suffering or other undesired conditions in life. This may be voluntary, involuntary or non-voluntary, and carried out with or without a physician. In a medical environment, this can be carried out by oral, intravenous, or intra-muscular drug administration.

Laws around the world vary greatly with regard to euthanasia and are constantly subject to change as cultural values shift and better palliative care or treatments become available. It is legal in some nations, while in others it may be criminalized. Due to gravity of the issue, strict restrictions and proceedings are enforced regardless of legal status. Euthanasia is a controversial issue because of conflicting moral feelings both for the individual and between different cultures, ethnicities, religions and other groups. The subject is explored by the mass media, authors, film makers and philosophers, and is the source of ongoing debate and emotion.

Let us analyse three different types of euthanasia :

1. *Voluntary Euthanasia* : Most of the groups campaigning for changes in the law to allow euthanasia are campaigning for voluntary euthanasia, ie., euthanasia carried out at the request of the person killed. Sometimes voluntary euthanasia is sacredly distinguishable from assisted suicide. Dr. Jack Kevorkian, a Michigan pathologist went on to build a 'suicide machine' to help terminally ill people commit suicide. Euthanasia can be voluntary if a person, while in good health, makes a written request for euthanasia if, through accident or illness, he/she should come to be incapable of making or expressing a decision to die, in pain, or without the use of her mental faculties, and there is no reasonable hope of recovery. Netherlands is the only country where doctors can openly help their patients to die in a peaceful and dignified way. In Netherlands, a series of court cases during the 1980s uphold a doctor's right to assist a patient to die. It has been estimated that about 2,300 deaths each year result from euthanasia carried out in this way.
2. *Involuntary Euthanasia* : Euthanasia may be regarded as involuntary when the person killed is capable of consenting to her/his own death, but does not do so, either because she/he is not asked or because when asked chooses to go on living. However there is significant difference between killing someone who chooses to go on living and killing someone who has not consented to being killed, but if asked, would have consented.
3. *Non-voluntary Euthanasia* : If a human being is not capable of understanding the choice between life and death, euthanasia would be neither voluntary nor involuntary but non-voluntary. Those unable to give consent would include

> incurably ill or severely disabled infants, and people who through accident, illness, or old age have permanently lost the capacity to understand the issue involved, without having previously requested or rejected euthanasia in these circumstances.

The case of someone who has never been capable of choosing to live or die is a little more straight forward than that of a person who had but now lost, the capacity to make such a decision. If we were to approach the issue of life or death for a seriously disabled human infant without any prior discussion of the ethics of killing in general, we might be unable to resolve the conflict between the widely accepted obligation to protect the sanctity of human life, and the goal of reducing suffering. Some say that such decisions are 'subjective' or that life and death questions must be left to God and Nature. It has been argued against killing human being because he is rational, autonomous and self-conscious being. Infants lack these characteristics. Killing them, therefore, cannot be equated with killing normal human beings or any other self-conscious beings. This conclusion is not limited to infants, who, because of irreversible intellectual disabilities, will never be rational, self-conscious beings. However one important reason why it is normally a terrible thing to kill an infant, is the effect the killing will have on its parents. It is different when the infant is born with a serious disability. Parents may with good reason, regret that the death of the child will have on its parents, can be a reason for rather than against killing it. In such cases, the parents of such infants should be able to make decision.

Under existing laws in most countries, people suffering unavoidable pain or distress from an incurable illness who beg their doctors to end their lives are asking their doctors to risk a murder charge. Although juries are extremely reluctant to convict in cases of this kind, the law is clear that neither the request, nor the degree of suffering, nor the incurable condition of the persons killed, is a defense to a charge of murder. Advocates of voluntary euthanasia propose that this law be changed so that a doctor could legally act on a patient's desire to die without further suffering.

Let us consider the difference between euthanasia and wilful death or suicide and analyze the views of philosophers regarding suicide. We have to observe whether it is lawful to kill oneself. Analyzing the problem of suicide we find that it is undoubtedly reflected upon by most individuals at some time in their lives, either when they themselves are in period of anxiety or depression or when news of suicide comes to them. The special qualities of the act of suicide are finality and ultimacy: for the suicide one commits is an act which is final because it cannot be undone and which is ultimate (as far as earthly life is concerned at least) because it destroys the basis human consciousness, for any and all meaning and value.

Here we are required to clarify that not all taking (or giving) one one's life is normally considered suicide. Even ethical theories which teach principles of self-directed action and development can include reference to giving one's life for others or sacrificing one's life when such is the highest value of which one is capable. Thus, a war hero who falls on a grenade to take his company or the donor of a kidney who subsequently dies is not usually considered a suicide. Suicide is an individual-centred, life-taking act whose motive is ceasing the struggle for values and resigning the search for meaning. Mention of motives suggests a number of issues that are raised by a study of suicide. Chief among them are the worth of life itself, the 'justification of that worth and the control over individual life that one ought to have'. Decisions about value as are involved in the problem of worth of life. Is life itself a value? Is it an intrinsic value or is it solely instrumental? Concerning these questions Seneca (4 B.C. 65 A.D.) suggests that not life but the quality or value of life is the important matter. He, therefore, believes that reason, as man's capacity for determining quality, can at certain times advise us to dic. Augustine finds no authority for suicide, nor he believes does suicide ever indicate any greatness of spirit. Extending Augustine's view, Aquinas maintains that suicide is related to the natural law tradition of ethics. He too finds that life, as a God-given gift, is to be prized as a value and that its willful cessation is always an evil.

Augustine and Aquinas refer to moral principle. Life for them has the value it does because of the ultimate belief that all being (and, therefore, all good) derives from God. A very different principle is found in the writing of David Hume, one of the great representatives of social utilitarianism. Hume fails to find away valid religious, legal, or moral argument against suicide, and concludes that suicide may be consistent with, even useful for, the good of society as well as of self. Modern philosopher Schopenhauer uses roughly the same sort of principle as Hume in considering the value of suicide, yet he draws a rather different conclusion. After reviewing a number of opinions on suicide, he finds that anxiety may indeed compel one to break off with life. But suicide remains a very clumsy act, for it abolishes the consciousness which should be aware of the cessation of the anxieties it is to accomplish.

One another major problem, i.e., problem of moral obligation, whether suicide is ever right, Seneca, establishes that under certain circumstances reason can advise or oblige us to die. As far as the theologians like St. Augustine and St. Aquinas are concerned they strongly reject the above view and instead support the protection of life. Regarding moral obligation, Hume believes that the principle of usefulness to self or society may sometimes make it right to commit suicide, but schopenhauer finds suicide clumsy, if not exactly morally wrong. William James, the great American pragmatist. and Albert Camus, great existentialist, make subtle analyses of the problem of obligation. James finds that the worth of living (as against dying) and the consequent obligation to live are not so much 'givens' as accomplishments by believing and living with these convictions, we can product or bring about the value and the obligation. Finally, Camus, reflecting existentialist themes, observes that suicide is not a form of revolt as some would have it, but it is rather an ultimate acceptance of the 'absurd' (the threat of meaninglessness) and death. Yet, he says revolt is what gives life its meaning—indeed, revolt in the presence of the absurd gives life all the purpose and value it has. Thus we can generalize that the idealists, theists and theologians regard that it is not lawful for man to take his own life whereas the sophists, utilitarian and to a large extent, the existentialists favour taking one own's life if it is not worth living.

From above discussion it is clear that taking one's own life or opting wilful death is not always unlawful or sin. In special circumstances cessation of life can be supported. As far as the justification of voluntary euthanasia is concerned, being well-thought rational decision of a self-conscious autonomous human being, it can be justified with certain conditions, which may be mentioned in the following manner :

- It is carried out by a physician.
- The patient has explicitly requested euthanasia in a manner that leaves no doubt of the patient's desire to die.
- The patient has an irreversible condition causing protracted physical or mental suffering that the patients find unbearable.
- There is no reasonable alternative (reasonable form the patient's point of view) to alleviate the patients suffering.
- The doctor has consulted another independent professional who agrees with his or her judgement. Euthanasia in these circumstances can be strongly supported and demand for law regarding it should be framed by the government to make it legal.

NOTES

Ethical Choice, Robert N. Beck, & John B. Orr (A Case Study Approach). The Tree Press (A division of MacMillan Publishing Co., New York, Collier MacMillan Publishers, London, (1970).

The City of God, St. Augustine, trans by John Healy Dulton & Co., Inc. and J.M. De Sons Ltd., Vol. 2.

The Myth of Sisphus, Albert Camus, trans. by Justin O, Brien. Alfred A. Knopt, Inc. Hamish Hamilton, London.

The Philosophical Works of David Hume, Boston-Little, Broon David.

Practical Ethics, Peter Singer, Cambridge University Press, 1993.

Selected Essays, Arthor Sehopenhauer Ernest Belfort Box (London) George Belt & Sons., 1909).

Summa Theologica - Thomas Aquinas, New York : Enziger Brothers, Inc. : London, Burns & Oaks Ltd., 1957.

Chapter 6

Cloning : Some Ethical Issues

Jyotish Ch. Basak

Much before cloning had emerged as a tangible actuality achieved by scientists, the human mind, by virtue of its ability to visualize and fantasize had toyed with the idea and painted a picture of the possible consequences which would occur if cloning became a reality. Therefore, many of ours attitudes and positions were born out of our understanding derived from these sources, which invariably revolved around situations in which untethered and unmonitored application of cloning had been done. The importance of understanding the implications of such situations is very great because science fiction is the product of brainstorming, in which ideas come out free and spontaneous. These may appear improbable at one point of time but may become distinct possibilities at some other. Taking cognizance of such dangers helps man to evolve a suitable framework and system of inbuilt safeguards within which the functioning of various endeavours should be contained.

However, equally important is the fact that an objective, dispassionate view, which takes account of merits and usefulness, should be taken. Many aspects of this scientific achievement contain potentials for the welfare and well-being of mankind. The application of genetic cloning for the understanding and control of disease that is, therapeutic cloning is one such aspect. Focussing on the possibility of achieving better understanding at the molecular level and thus on more effective treatment and control, one finds optimistic evidence in the area of genetic cloning.

Many government conducted heated debates (in the Indian Parliament too there was a debate about this) on these issues. However, if one goes through the proceedings, one finds that commercial interests of certain influential organizations were predominantly echoed in statements made rather than an evaluation of the intrinsic issues. And considering that a large amount of money is involved, and the power of money is unbelievably strong, no one can hold back the tide. The only alternative at our disposal is to evolve an ethically viable framework and parameter within which the enterprise should grow, so that value based science triumphs over the rat race for money.

The History of Cloning

The concept of cloning has not come all at once. It took long time for people to realize this process and coining the term. Early humans discovered that if they plant seeds produced by the healthiest plants, the next crop will be a stronger one. This discovery of better breed of corn was perhaps the first step in manipulating life to suit human needs. Thousands of years later to ease their backbreaking labour, we find the farmers breeding female horses with male asses to produce mules (mules were desirable beasts of burden because of their endurance, surefootedness, intelligence and long lifespan). Much later in 1952 a tiny tadpole makes history as the first cloned animal. Using cells from a tadpole embryo, Robert Briggs and Thomas King created new tadpoles identical to the original donor. Soon after that there was a rapid development one after another. In 1965, cloning goes to box office in the movie *classic, THE HUMAN DUPLICATORS*. Primitive special effects dominate this hilarious alien-invaders flick. In 1972, cloning steeped down to the micro level with the first cloning of a gene. Scientists , isolated the gene, and then bound it to an organism (in this instance an yeast) that incorporated the gene into its own DNA and multiplied, producing many copies of the desired gene. In 1976, Rudoff Janeisch of the Salk Institute for Biological Studies in La Jolla, California, injected human DNA into newly fertilised mouse eggs to produce mice that are part of human. When the mice reproduced, they passed their human genetic material to their offsprings, creating a slew of so-called transgenic mice. Different human diseases could be studied by creating mice with the appropriate genetic combination. In 1978, the world for the first time listened to the news of first test-tube baby. The world clamoured for a glimpse of Baby Louise, the first child conceived through in vitro fertilization (using the husband's sperm, British doctors fertilised an egg in a petri dish, then implanted the embryo in the uterus of the healthy woman). In 1978, David Rorvik's published his *In His Image*: The *Cloning of a Man.* In the novel, a man is cloned from skin cells. In 1987, the first mammals, sheep and cows, were cloned from embryonic cells. But animals cloned from embryonic cells contain the genetic material of both parents because the embryos are sexually fertilised. Clones from embryonic cells from the same parents different times are as different as brothers and sisters. In 1993, the episode of Dinosaur cloning appeared in super movie Jurassic Park A few strands of historic DNA have fossiled, and that was enough for an ambitious park owner to wreck genetic havoc. In 1995, sequencing all of a bacterium's genetic material was accomplished by J. Craig Venter of the Institute for Genomic Research in Rockville. Venter uses chemical analysis to identify all the genes of *Hemophilus influenzae,* the bacterium that causes meningitis and children's ear infection. Scientists hoped to sequence the human genome by 2005 (but completed much ahead of deadline), which would enable scientists to target specific genes for research.

In 1996, Dolly was cloned but the world did not know until 1997, when her existence was revealed. Using older techniques as well as some new tricks, Scottish researcher Ian Wilmut cloned Dolly from an adult cell.

The birth of Dolly has an extraordinary impact on many dimensions of our lives, both intellectual and real. It has fuelled debate on a number of issues: genetic, scientific, political, moral, journalistic, and literary. It has also given rise to a number of myths, not least among which is the myth that Dolly presents a danger to humanity, the human gene-poll, genetic diversity the ecosystem, the world, as we know it, and the survival of human species.

There was an amazing spontaneous reaction after the disclosure of the news. The reaction of the scientific community was, on the whole, friendly. In contrast, the reaction of the public at large was overwhelmingly negative, primed to some extent by a media weaned on a diet of previous cloning scares stories and pulp fiction. People all around the world felt that something morally problematic was threatening to happen. Most of the concern Centres not on the cloning of sheep, but on the likelihood that sooner or later someone will clone a human being.

In the following sections our effort will be to look at the current debate, the benefits and concerns about cloning. Cloning offers a useful starting-point for those who need convenient access to information about the many issues involved in genetic engineering. Let us start with the basic question: what is human cloning? We need to know this because non-understanding of it gives rise to much confusion.

What is Human Cloning?

Human cloning is the creation of a human being, or a number of human beings, who is/are genetically identical to the donor. In the current debate, we usually hear Cloning referred to in one of two ways: *Reproductive Cloning* and *Therapeutic Cloning. Reproductive Cloning* refers to the creation of a new person with the same genetic make-up as someone who is alive or has lived. *Therapeutic cloning* refers to using cloning techniques to initiate the growth of embryos in order to create new organs or cells for medical and research purpose.

Artificial cloning can be carried out by one of two techniques: Embryo splitting and nuclear replacement. *Embryo splitting is* similar to the natural process which creates identical twins —the embryo's cells are separated at a very early stage of development to create one or more clones. *Nuclear replacement* is the process that was used to create Dolly, the sheep. It works by taking a cell nucleus from one person (e.g., from a skin cell) and putting it into the egg of another, whose nucleus has already been removed. The egg is then stimulated to divide, for example, by treatment with bursts of electric current, thus starting the growth of an embryo. The egg's nucleus contains all the chromosomes (genetic information) for the cell to start dividing and become a fully developed child in due course. Nuclear replacement technology can be used to create a clone from a person of any stage (embryo, foetus or adult), and it can potentially create many more clones than embryo splitting.

Cloning seems to offer new possibilities of medical advances. Some people might want to use cloning to replace a dead baby or child; or indeed have a child if they are infertile. Others may want to replicate themselves for future generations, while yet others may want to create a clone to produce an organ for transplantation without complications of rejecting the organ, i.e., for therapeutic purposes.

How did People React to the News

As soon as the news of cloning Dolly broke out, almost every organisation and every sensitive person reacted to it. On the one hand, there were those that felt that fits and advances gained from cloning outweighed any social dilemmas; on that other hand, there were those that felt that cloning is wrong on a fundamental moral level and would produce scientific and social problems. In weighing these views, major organisations drew on numerous sources including religious law, party philosophy and scientific concerns. Some objected to cloning on a purely ethical level, while others favoured cloning solely for the scientific advances it would produce. Let us state here some of the stances of some prominent religious, scientific, and ethical groups.

From the Catholic Church John Paul-II released a statement condemning the cloning of all life forms. The Vatican also issued a statement that only condemned human cloning, but did not address other forms. Martin Robra, executive secretary, the World Council of Churches commented that the Council would prefer a moratorium until all ethical questions could be resolved. Marry Seller, from Church of England Board of Social Responsibility, commented: 'The antics of a few cranks and Hitler types' should not impede cloning research. 'Cloning, like all sciences, must be used responsibly. Cloning humans is not desirable. But cloning sheep has its uses.'

Islamic scholars took an ambivalent attitude towards this scientific advancement. Abdelmo'ti Bayyumi, a theologian from Al-Azhar University, declared it is forbidden to clone animals under Islamic law. However, some Muslim scholars testified to the National Bioethics Advisory Committee that they felt that cloning might be allowable if it produced ways to counteract infertility.

The chief Rabbi of Israel, Meir Law, stated that the cloning of any creature is against Jewish law. However, some Jews believe that cloning in order to produce better food and medication would be allowable in Jewish tradition.

Different scientific and economic organisations were by and large in favour of accepting this new-found technology, of course, with safeguards. Stephen Grebe, Professor of Biology, American University said: "We're going to be facing this issue with humans.... With that possibility open, I'm concerned that without safeguards this will become a reality. Randolfe Wicker, founder of Clones Rights United Front, said: "We're fighting for research, and we're defending people's reproductive rights." Steve Dasch, Chairman of the Libertarian Party writes: "Politican should not have veto power over the creation of new life—especially human life....That's why the Libertarian Party supports reproductive freedom of choice — whether they choose to reproduce using traditional method, or artificial insemination or in vitro fertilisation, or cloning ... if, arch is banned, millions of people could suffer". On the other side of the table we have Jeremy Rifkin, President, Foundation of Economic Trends. Proposing a world-wide ban on cloning, he says it should carry a penalty 'on par with rape, child abuse and murder'.

Carl Felbaum, President of Biotechnology Industry Organisation, says: "One of the prospects should not be, perhaps, should never be, the extension of this technique to human beings ... Now that it may be possible we would say it should be prohibited if necessary by law".

These observations reveal a reservation against human cloning.

Law on Cloning

- In the Indian Parliament the possibility of cloning was discussed. But it was declared by the concerned Minister that there was no possibility of cloning in the near future on the Indian soil. Hence, there was no need of bringing a bill for banning cloning.
- In the West, in March 1997, the European Parliament voted in a resolution to ban cloning of human beings. However, the resolution carries no legal weight. This cloning of human being policy area remains more obviously a matter for individual member states, with national politicians bringing in legislation on human cloning.
- In December 1997, UNESCO published the Universal Declaration on the Human Genome and Human Rights. Article 11 bans 'practices which are contrary to human dignity, such as reproductive cloning of human beings...'
- In Strasbourg, the Council of Europe, with 40 member states, produced a protocal banning human cloning which has been added to their Convention on Biomedicine and Human Rights, and was signed on 12 January, 1998 by 19 member states.

The U.K. Government rejecting expert advice blocked any move to clone human for the production of tissue for transplants and a range of other medical score mongering. The pro-cloning group accused the government of giving in to media. Some Governments also rejected the recommendation that cloning embryos for the supply of cells, and tissue for medicine should be allowed. Scientists claimed that therapeutic cloning would harness the techniques used to clone Dolly, the sheep, to turn a cell from a patient into compatible tissue and cells for transplant. However, Government said that more evidence was needed — from animal research, for instance for its potential benefits to human health.

Despite governmental legislation of blocking human cloning researchers were confident that despite a hiatus, human tissue will be grown soon. A government frightened by public resentment of genetically modified foods was hardly likely to push its luck with something that, would be presented as approval for human cloning. Such attitudes call for a consideration of the misconceptions about cloning.

Some Misconceptions about Cloning

Most cloning misconceptons arise from a lack of knowledge. Most people do not understand the basic principles of cloning, and are likely to make rash generalisations about whether cloning is natural or not: Other misconceptions focus on the societal problems resulting from cloning. Many of these misconceptions are only valid in a society where the laws are slack or are not properly enforced. People forget that along with new technological developments come rules and guidelines to prevent the kind of scenarios here. Each misconception results from a distortion of the truth, which is presented here, with each incorrect belief.

- A clone would not be a normal human.
- Cloning is 'playing God'.
- Cloning is not a natural process.
- Clone will not have a soul.
- A clone will have the same feelings and emotions as its genetic parent.
- An unconscious clone could be produced to supply organs.
- Someone could own a clone.
- Great individuals of the past could be reproduced.

As to the first point (i.e., a clone would not be a normal human) let us say that *whatever the* methods of reproduction, a clone would be as 'human' as an identical twin. Both are derived from a single fertilized egg.

About the second point let me make it clear that cloning does not create life, as this stigma implies. Cloning merely produces life from existing life. Cloning can be thought of as an extension of procedures like *in vitro* fertilisation.

It is not true that cloning is not a natural process. Cloning utilises elements that already exist in the natural reproduction process. Embryo cloning pulls apart a zygote at the two-cell stage and creates two one-celled organisms. Some might say that cloning is not intended form of reproduction, the same might be said of *in vitro* fertilisation, and the use of fertility drugs.

The fourth point seems to imply that the soul is a quantifiable physical element of someone's genetic make-up, that is, it can be altered or taken away. In this case, cloning does not present more of a religious problem than identical twins. Despite there being identical, it is agreed that both twins have souls.

It is a myth, say experts, that a "clone will have the same feelings and emotions as its genetic parent. An oft-taken example of this idea is a Hitler clone starting a new Holocaust. While genes and genetic structure can give certain characteristics and emotional tendencies, environment and upbringing play a much larger role in shaping someone's emotions and outlook. A Hitler clone that had been raised shaping somewhere else and had lived in a period of stability and prosperity would not act in the same way as a Hitler raised in Germany living amongst post-war devastation and hatred.

About the next point we may say that despite being morally questionable, producing a clone with no self-awareness requires a deeper knowledge of where the consciousness resides. Consciousness is not certainly a trait that can be erased through genetics, and there can be no isolated DNA that determines its existence. Furthermore, just proving that a clone is not self-aware would be difficult. People with debilitating neurological disorders may appear mentally incapacitated but retain full consciousness. However, researchers have theorised the possibility of cloning only certain organs to be used as replacements, in dire need of an individual for transplant. Scientists believe that if the cells of an organ have the same genetic make-up as those of the host organism, the organ would be much less likely to be rejected after a transplant.

Although cloning is being considered as a future infertility remedy, and essentially, a clone would be made for the parents, no one could own a clone. Ownership of a clone would be no different than slavery. People that predict a massive working underclass produced from cloning forget that despite the methods of their birth, clones would carry the same rights' as a person produced through normal reproduction.

About the final point, all current techniques to clone an adult cell use the method of nuclear transfer, which requires the donor cell to be alive. In this process a live adult cell is fused with an egg cell or its nucleus is extracted and inserted into the egg. At this time, and most likely far into the future, clones of dead organisms cannot be created. Also, even if such an individual is cloned, the development of the person is dependent upon its upbringing and childhood surroundings. Just as a Hitler clone would most likely not grow up to start a new Holocaust, an Einstein clone would probably not become a world renowned physicist.

Benefits of Cloning

There are many ways in which human cloning is expected to benefit mankind. Here is a list which is far from complete.

- It may some day be possible to reverse the ageing process because of what we learn from cloning.
- Scientists believe that they may be able to treat heart-attack victims by cloning their healthy heart cells and injecting them into the areas of the heart that have been damaged. Heart disease, we know, is the number one killer in many countries.

- Embryonic stem cells can be grown to produce organs or tissues to repair or replace damaged ones. Skin for burn victims, brain cells for the brain damaged, hearts, lungs, livers, and kidneys could be produced. By combining this technology with human cloning technology it may be possible to produce needed tissue for suffering people. Such tissue will be free of rejection by their immune systems. Many diseases will become curable if human cloning and its technology are not banned.
- With cloning, infertile couples could have children. Despite getting a fair amount of publicity in the news, current treatments for infertility, in terms of percentage, are not very successful. Couples go through physically and emotionally painful procedures for a small chance of having children. Many couples run out of time and money without any success at having children. Human cloning could make it possible for many more infertile couples to have children than ever before.
- Because of human cloning and its technology, the days of silicone breast implants and other cosmetic procedures that may cause immune disease should soon be over. With new technology, instead of using materials foreign to the body for such procedures, doctors will be able to manufacture bone, fat, connective tissue, or cartilage that matches the patient's tissues exactly. Anyone will be able to have them altered to their satisfaction without the leaking of silicon gel into the other problems that occur with present-day plastic surgery. Victims of terrible accidents that deform their features should now be able to have them repaired with new and safer technology.
- The average person carries eight defective genes inside them. These defective genes allow people to become sick when they would otherwise remain healthy. With human cloning and its technology it may be possible to ensure that we no longer suffer because of our defective genes.

- We may learn how to switch cells on and off through cloning and thus be able to cure cancer. Scientists still do not know exactly how cells differentiate into specific kinds of tissue, nor do they understand why cancerous cells lose their differentiation. Cloning, at long last, may be the key to understanding differentiation and cancer.
- Cloning technology can be used to test and perhaps cure genetic diseases.

The above list only scratches the surface of what human cloning technology can do for mankind. The suffering that can be relieved is staggering. This new technology heralds a new era of unparalleled advancement in medicine if people are released from their fears and let the benefits begin. Why should another child die from leukemia when, if the technology is allowed, we should be able to cure it in a few years time?

Until the birth of Dolly; it was believed that the ability to clone an adult human was either impossible or possible only in the distant future. However, human embryos have been twinned in the past. These were true clones but they were not viable, however, for they did not survive.

The emergence of new technologies creates a new set of cultural events and their consequences with which human cultures must come to terms. Humans must define a status and a role of any new technology. This is a process of adaptation and acculturation. In a sense, this is a process whereby humans try to decide what a new 'means' to them. Questions frequently asked during this process of acculturation and adaptation include:

- What are the needs and goals this technology might serve? Is this technology the only means for addressing these goals and needs?
- What members of which communities have these goals and needs?
- Of these groups in need who will have access to the

technology and its products; for example will it be only special individuals or classes of people?

- Who will be benefited, and who will be harmed, indirectly as well as directly, by implementation of this new technology?
- How reliable, how safe, and how well can this new technology be controlled?
- What is the best case, and what is the worst case, scenario if this technology were encouraged, or if it were impeded, in its development and implementation?
- Is this new technology to be defined as 'necessary' or 'essential', or 'innocuous' or "superfluous" or 'good' or 'bad'?
- Is this technology, or are its consequences, to be deemed ethical, moral, immoral?
- Should this technology be considered a form of 'property', to be held by individuals or publicly held and administered? And if so, by whom?

Should Humans be Cloned?

God cloned Eve as there was a necessity for Him to create a woman and a wife for Adam. If it is right for God, how could it be wrong for humans to do the same thing? But in reality, it may be unethical for humans to clone anything, including humans, when he has been provided the perfect mechanism for propagation, like having babies with love and passion. Cloning of an adult to an adult is beyond the knowledge of humans as of this day. From this point alone, cloning to have babies may not be all that ethical unless there are other reasons to justify this method. Anything that cannot be justified is unethical. The cloning science is exact, whereas the ethics part of it is subjective, and subjective issues are dictated by people who have resources to implement their wills over the society. All the ethical conduct that we see around us may not be at all that ethical if the rationality and truthfulness had prevailed without hindrance.

A Times Magazine poll (March 10, 1997) reported that 74 per cent of those asked believe, it is against God's will to clone human beings. President Clinton has banned federal funds from being used for human cloning research, stating that: "Any discovery that touches upon human creation is not simply a matter of scientific inquiry, it is a matter of morality and spirituality as well... Each human life is unique, born of a miracle that reaches beyond laboratory science..."

But others argue in favour of continuing human cloning research, of continuing to clone human embryos and perhaps cloning adult humans in the future. Some arguments in favour of human cloning might include the fact that cloned human embryos would make research into genetics and genetically related diseases, and their treatments or preventions, much easier and cheaper. Cloning embryos could also facilitate the process of *in vitro* fertilisation, since the collection and replacement of ova is often painful and traumatic, and can be unsuccessful.

We have already mentioned that embryo cloning is seen as a potential treatment for infertility when *in vitro* fertilisation is not available, such as when parents are infertile, or when one or both parents harbours a genome coding for certain undesirable traits or diseases, or if the parents are homosexual couples. Cloned embryonic tissues might be used for the replacement of lost or diseased tissues.

Adult cloning might appeal to those who desire children/adults who are genetically identical to themselves, or genetically identical to someone who is a nonfamily member. Cloning could provide a genetically identical replacement far a lost loved one.

Perhaps the most urgent ethical, legal and social issues about cloning arise in the end-process that may lead to the birth of a first human clone. This is so because, as has been pointed out by scholars, early human experiments are likely to result in a number of clinical failures and lead to miscarriage, the necessity of dozens or even hundred of abortions, or births of massively deformed offspring. Recent study of mammalian cloning also suggests that a number of defects often created in the reprogramming of the egg do not manifest themselves until later in the life of the resulting clone, so that mature clones have often undergone spectacular, unforeseen deaths.

The dangers for early prospective clones are controversial and difficult to manage because.

- In part, one is attempting to protect a future potential person against harms that might be inflicted by their very existence, and
- In part because societies around the world have indicated that they believe that the early cloning experiments will breach a natural barrier that is moral in character, taking humans into a realm of self-engineering that vastly exceeds any prior experiments with new reproductive technology.

Human Cloning from Religious Perspectives

The most commonly cited ethical and moral arguments against human cloning seem to originate from religious perspective. These religious arguments can even be made by politicians and scientists with religious sympathies. Many religious philosophies teach, for example, that human life is unique and special and should be created, determined and controlled' only by their deities. Many religions believe in the existence of, and in the individuality of, a human soul. Many Christians, for example, will be concerned about whether it will be possible to clone the human soul, along with the human. If it is possible tc clone the soul, what will this mean? In contrast, if a person is cloned, but not their soul, what will this mean? Can a clone without a soul be and not offend our moral and religious beliefs?

Not all religious leaders, of course, feel the same. In contrast to the opinions of their peers, some Jewish and Muslim religious leaders testified before the National Bioethics Advisory Commission that they feel that embryo and cloning research might provide discoveries that would lead to an appropriate way to counter infertility.

Is Human Cloning scientifically ethical?

Currently, human cloning is illegal in many countries. In the U.S., federal, but not private, funds are prohibited from being used to create human embryos or do research on human embryos if they will be harmed or destroyed. In addition, the then President Clinton imposed a moratorium on human cloning research. As, decision makers in various countries debate whether or not to support research on human embryos and human cloning, many ethical and legal questions arise.

For example, how will the state ban on human cloning research and the ban on certain types of human embryo research affect other, related fields of research that are deemed important? Human embryo and human cloning research can be used to conduct research and development of contraceptives, studies aimed at understanding the causes of human infertility and its solutions, research involving genetic testing, genetic engineering, disease diagnosis, prevention and treatment, and in testing various medicines and medical procedures. In contrast, if the government funds this type of research, then it will have some important control over the nature of the research. If the government decides to continue to not fund human embryo and cloning research, then the government will not have one important avenue for controlling, to some degree; the nature of the research. If the government refuses to support this research, would a funding vacuum be left that market forces will quickly fill? If the private sector is left to fund research and development, then will this research be driven by entrepreneurial profit motives? What effects will entrepreneurial forces have on the nature of such research and development?

Another related question is: Does the governmental ban violate academic freedom and the right to think, inquire, and do research? When or should the research involving human embryos and cloning be defined as 'academic research and inquiry'? If this research is defined as academic, should the scientific research on human embryos and cloning be protected under the guarantees of 'freedom of speech'? Here there are limits to the kinds of speech that is protected under the above freedom. For example, it does not protect speech that is deemed to be obscene, or speech deemed threatening to national security. Some citizens believe that research into and/or trying to clone humans is wrong; while others disagree. When considering whether or not cloning research, or other kinds of academic research, inquiry, and scientific communication are to be protected, and to what degree, by the above freedom, the government decision makers have to decide how best to balance protecting the freedoms of speech and inquiry of the scientific community— and benefits their research might produce— against the need to protect other citizens from any dangers of this kind of freedom of speech, and its products, might also produce.

In the absence of governmental controls, can/or should the scientific community regulate itself, through peer review; when it comes to human embryo and cloning research? Should society entrust the scientific community to regulate themselves? Would this allow and encourage practices leading to conflicts of interest? Should some other private organisation, independent of the scientific community or the federal government, have this responsibility?

Finally, and perhaps more importantly, if there is a market for human embryo and cloning research, and the products of their research, can any type of legislation, at any level, aimed at restricting them be effectively enforced?

A democracy is designed to facilitate a balance between competing interests, to achieve the maximum benefit for the maximum number of its citizens. The introduction of new technology challenges a democratic society to decide who gets what, when, where and how much. The advent of cloning *via* nuclear transfer technology presents the inevitability of new and important social changes, and new issues concerning this power.

Another important questions is: What do genetic engineering, and the cloning of human beings, mean for sociological and legal definitions of, and concepts concerning, the notions of 'individual', 'human', and 'citizenship'? These will be some of the most difficult and interesting questions that need to be decided. Would a cloned human be an individual? Would it really be a human, with a soul? And what if this clone were then cloned again, and again? What would their status and roles be? Would a non-human primate; such as chimpanzee, who carried one or more human genes *via* transgenic technology, be defined as still a chimp, a human, a sub-human, or something else? If we choose to define it as a human, would we then have to give it rights of citizenship? And if humans were to carry non-human, transgenic genes, *would that* alter our definitions and treatments of them?

Another important issues is eugenics. Can we, and should we, use the biotechnologies of genetic manipulation and cloning to improve the human condition? What are some of the perceived risks and benefits of eugenics? Other questions and issues include a revitalisation of the 'nature/nurture' debate. Will cloned humans really look exactly alike? Will they have identical personalities? How will clones impact the future of twin studies meant to ferret out the different impacts of genes *vs*. the environment? What will human clones be able to contribute to the perspectives of sociobiology?

Hilary Putnam argues that cloning humans violates human dignity even when the purpose is not as blatantly instrumental as producing an organ donor. For him, the issue poses an extremely grave problem. The problem may be for two reasons: (1) the scenario that we learn how to clone people, and (2) the technology becomes widely employed, not just by infertile couples, but by ordinary fertile people who simply wish to have a child just like so-and-so. Putnum is of the view that there are many grounds, including some obvious grounds, for being worried about the possible misuse of cloning technology. For Putnum, before deciding the fate of technology what we need first and foremost is a moral image of the world. Write Ruth Anna Putnum, without a moral image any moral philosophy is incomplete. In his book *The Many Faces of Realism* he defines moral image not as a declaration that this or that is a virtue or a right, it is rather a picture of how our virtues and ideals hang together with one another, and what they have to do with the position we are in. We can get a richer appreciation of the Kantian project in ethics if we see the detailed principles that Kant argued for as flowing from such a moral image (an image of human equality). Unlike Kant, Putnum favours a *plurality* of moral images. In his plurality of images Putnum conceives some moral images of the family, moral images which turn out to influence how we think not *just* about the family but about communal life in general. We do use images derived from family life in structuring our whole way of looking at society and our whole way of seeing our moral responsibilities to one another. This is a crucial point of view. This view amounts in fact to saying that we live in a moral community defined by certain basic moral concepts and principles. The question of good and bad technology cannot be decided in isolation from the question whether it seriously undermines our moral image of the world, threatens to undermine it or erodes the bond of association that holds it together.

Chapter 7

Human Cloning : Some Bioethical Questions

D.N. Tiwari

The technological era of ours has compelled us to accept that man can't live not only without techniques but even without technology also because it, in new millennium, man has got an inevitable place into the very structure not only of our social but of our cultural life also. Technology has almost become the synonym of our entire advancement influencing ways of life and, the life style of the people of the millennium. The technological society of ours, unlike the nineteenth century European industrial society, considers that machines segregate man from society but technology integrates machines with society. Machines, when integrated with society, help us in getting rid of our backwardness in different aspects of our lives. I am not going to push this issue in further detail and like to confine my reflections on the Bioethics of some technological inventions like human cloning.

The field and scope of bioethics are not fully defined as yet but one thing is very obvious that it includes the whole conduct of human person regarding the various ways of its behaviour with the life-world. Right to production, use and selling right of hybrid seeds and adrenals by multinational companies, Patent right of products of plants, shrubs, grains, right of blood donation, life preserving products, cruelty to animals for scientific and technological researches, hunting of rare birds and animals, destruction of rare lives on the earth, preservation of human excellence, pesticide, foeticide, atomic garbage, sale of human organs, growth of population, sperm and egg banks, genetic transmutation, harvesting of stem cells, human clone and trade right of bio products are some very important issues which are burning topics of bioethical discussion of the present time.

However, it is clear that the aim and the basic ethics lying behind Biotechnology is to serve the humanity in a way to save the life of beings, to ensure the means so as to enable them to live a complete life span free from diseases and to preserve their capacity. Ultimately, its main objective is to save the rationality/wisdom and excellences on the earth.

Here, in this chapter, I confine my reflections to reveal the bioethical problems of human cloning and even so with few instances from our scriptures.

It is evident from the scriptures that Vedic India was highly developed in the field of spiritual knowledge and spiritual-technique but there is no historical evidence to accept that she was civilized more than the present world of science and technology. The seers considered the realization of spiritual powers assigned naturally to individuals as the supreme goal for the realization of which they sacrificed their whole life. It was the power of realization, which made them capable of knowing everything unknown to others. The spiritual techniques they invented for the welfare of the life on the earth were of more importance for the development and growth of human life, civilization and culture. As seers were of strong will and indefatigable devotion, it was not difficult for them to do anything successfully they willed. The successful accomplishment of anything implies restless concentration and methodical search without which doubt persists in finding the required result.

Modern scientists, of the continents other than Asia or even of Asia, may deny any influence of prehistoric inventions found in the scriptures and they may claim the originality of their inventions but it cannot be denied that technological achievements of today are prerequisitely progressively gradual in which the preceding inventions confer favour for progressive succeeding inventions. This may not be similar in case of prehistoric inventions of the seers that were new beginnings out of no material, no instrument or data available beforehand. They, as scriptures say, got the techniques as direct flashes of their super mental vision. Their vision is remarked as that in which the differences of subject and object are fused in a unity of the vision. A vision in which perceiver does not stand apart from and at a distance from the thing the identity and epistemological difference of both the subject and the object, at that moment, is transcended in the visionary concentration of truth which is neither a subject nor an object but knowledge itself. They practiced what they realized for the welfare of the life on the earth. Their experiences are preserved in the scriptures. Now-a-days, it is easy to understand that a serious researcher of any corner of the world keeps himself well aware of the informations belonging to any tradition and more than that it is not an exaggeration to say that the lives of those sacrificing themselves for the cause of scientific and technological inventions are not radically different from those of seers who sacrificed their lives for truth of the human persons and made it applicable to the welfare of them on the earth.

Cloning with some Instances from Indian Scriptures

In *Skandha* 9, *Adhyaya* 13, *Sl.* 13 of *Srimadbhagavat*, it has been mentioned that when his excellency Nimi was dead, the seers by process of Mantha, perhaps, human cloning in modern idioms, of his body created a new baby. The baby was called Janaka, as it was a birth out of cell of his father. It was called Videha, as it was not born from a mother but out of a non-sexual, non-conjugal process. As the baby was born out of a process of *mantha* it was called *Mithila* and his kingdom was named Mithila (*Janmana Janakah so'bhud vaidehastu videhajah, Mithilo mathanajjato mithila yena nirmita*). The questions arise; whether the *mantha kama* was the same that we know today by the word human cloning, whether the process adopted by the seers was the same that is applied by the technologists today and whether the ethics lying behind it was the same. I am unable to say anything on those questions except on the last because I have knowledge neither of *Mantha-karma* nor of human cloning. However, it is interesting to mention the morality lying behind *Mantha-karma* as the epic itself has specified it. The morality then was not to save the excellence and order only but to check the mayhem to be caused out of its deprivation also.

Proving the existence of God, Rene Descartes, a Rationalist Philosopher, gave an argument that man cannot make himself. Had he made himself he would have made him God. New technology of cloning has come with an imagination that man can make himself and even so in his own imagination.

Clone is a Greek term for twin identical, genetically and physically, from the male or female from which it is derived. The derivation of Dolly, a lamb by Dr. Ian Wihnot of Scotland, Neti and Ditho, kids of monkey, by Oregon Regional Primate Research Center of America have experimented that by transplanting D. N. A. of any animate, in ovary, clone can be prepared. The creation of animal clone paved the way for materialization of the fascination of technologicians to prepare clones.

Very recently, when I read in the newspapers that Advanced Cell Technology (ACT), a company of America, has prepared human clone by the name *'stem cell'*.

I recalled the epic story of hundred sons of Gandhari, the mother of Kauravas, born out of a stem cell prepared by the seer Veda Vyasa. Not only that but, the invention of 19 stem cell of human embryo by Advanced Cell Technology of America has also actualized the possibility of birth of 19 babies if all of them are implanted in separate 19 wombs. ACT is claiming that stem cells will be most useful for cure of diabetes, heart diseases, cancer, aids, loss of memory and inherited diseases. This advancement in clone technology is suspected as the beginning of the big plants of human clones. Not only Psychologists and Philosophers but also political, social and religious leaders have also started crying it immoral entombment of the natural order. I shall describe the bioethical issues of human cloning after few steps but before that I want to remark that it is by these inventions that we have come to believe that seer's speculations are myth is no longer but are truths that can be worked out even today by technological inventions.

Transplantation of Embryo

The first surgeon, in the history of human life, who successfully transplanted the embryo formed in the womb of Devaki, the mother of Krishna., the God of the epic *Mahabharata*, in the womb of Rohini, another wife of Vasudeva, the father of Krishna, was, as the epic says, a pre-historic she-deity named Yogamaya. *Srimadbhagavat Gita*, *adhyaya* 2, *skandha* 10. A revival of that pre -historic event is evidenced by the world recently with a successful transplantation of the embryo of a daughter in the womb of her mother by a team of doctors in U.S.A.

Rejuvenation

The story of old seer Cyavana enjoying juvenility even in very old age, as mentioned by Veda Vyasa in *Srimadbhagavad*, *adhyaya* 3, *skandha* 9, was considered, till very recently, only a myth but with recent technological invention of gene therapy by Dr. Lee Swine of University of Pennsylvania, has come to a truth.

As our body is completely controlled by genes any mutation or change in vitality of gene occurs in proportion to the increasing of age and, consequently, changes in muscles is naturally observed. These changes vary in case of our early years., adulthood and old age. If we allow the change of gene from early years to fifteenth of the age, as the maturity of mind takes place only up to fifteenth, and after that if we stop, for a possible period, the rate of change in gene, the duration of youthful years will be prolonged and, thus, the individual may achieve desired achievement of his life without feeling any fatigue and with all juvenility as well. This very mystery is successfully experimented by Dr. Lee through gene therapy.

Professor S.M. Hadi, of Department of Biochemistry, Aligarh Muslim University, Aligarh, in his paper entitled 'Recent Advances in Research on Ageing' presented at a National Seminar organized by the Department of Philosophy, AMU, Aligarh from February. 5-7,2002, expressed an altogether different view based on his experiment on house flies. According to his experiment there are cases of prolonged ageing if the issue belongs to one's later period of productive age. However, when asked he expressed doubt regarding certainty of his theory of ageing and accepted the theory of controlling mutation approximately at the age of fifteen years for ageing.

Technology, including Biotechnology, is value free; it is neither good nor evil in itself. It gets value as good or evil when associated or applied in society. For instance, the idea before the terminator gene technology was to yield best possible production of grains and, hence, it is valued as good but their distress was that the insects ate up their crops grown out of hybrid seeds and when they used pesticides they got their crops destroyed. We all know what happened to those farmers of the State of Andhra in India. They committed suicide out of distress not only of getting no production out of sowing the seeds produced by those hybrid seed crops, but of getting the soil deserted also.

This technology proved evil not only for them but for those who do not want to use those gene seeds but whose crops in the fields, close to the field with the crops using those seeds, are inflated due to open natural pollination, also. V.T. hybrid seeds replace those seeds but the farmers of the State are not allowed to use those seeds before well observed by the Government. In spite of all restrictions by the Government the poor farmers use those seeds for better crops and hence for benefits to earn more. What of the ethics?

The basic ethical idea, not only before the ancient inventions, as mentioned in the scriptures, but before the recent technological inventions also, is to preserve the excellence on one hand and to meet with threats that may cause anarchy and disorder in the society.

Advantage of Cloning

(a) Stem cell which is prepared by cloning, as claimed by technologicians, is the only fit remedy for getting rid not only of some of the diseases borrowed to one by heredity but for other diseases concerning cancer, heart, lung, liver, etc., in which replacement of healthy cells in the place of damaged cells are inevitably needed.

(b) Those pairs having no child will be privileged of getting a child out of the genetic material of their own by the cloning technology.

(c) Those pairs suffering from genetic diseases, which have made them physically and mentally incapable of getting birth of a child, may get relief by the human clone technology.

Cloning, from the scientific point of view, is a very splendid invention of the technology. It is a technological device and comes, in the society, with the ethics to preserve the life for great and sublime qualities/rationality on the earth on the one hand and to help remove our backwardness in the field of scientific knowledge on the other; and thus, it has a great value. But the question arises: cloning for what purpose? If, it is confined to grow human cells for cure of different inherited diseases, it must be welcome but if it is for creating a human clone for preserving some excellence, the question under consideration becomes more important. A task for the preservation of some excellence on the earth can't; ethically, be wrong. But it may be estimated useless, as even promoting gene technology may preserve the same. I don't know, only technologists know and can say, authentically, something about it. However, I propose to furnish few comments of my own on it after few paragraphs but before that I want to say that human cloning when evaluated connectedly with society we, apart from its all-scientific and technological importance, find it not only paradoxical but with nothing to live for also. Here below, I am giving reasons, given from different point of views but related to the ethical issue of human cloning, for proving my statement.

Deformation of Human Nature

(a) Human being is a unique combination of rationality and animality. If, in the process of nurturing the clone, of a male, after and before its transplantation in the womb of a women, the excess of Y chromosomes are artificially destroyed in order to balance the desired proportion of both of the chromosomes bearing supra and infra qualities, undoubtedly, super excellent super rational beings, will be born but then they will be deprived of those excellence to be acquired by a mother. Not only that but he wilI be a particular excellence of a person of which it is a clone. In such a circumstance, it will not be different from a machine or a particular excellence and, thus, there is a possibility of destruction and deviation of rest of the qualities by that of particular quality.

(b) There must be danger of losing self-identity of clones also. It will be difficult to differentiate not only the clone from the person of which it is a clone but several clones of the same person also, if they appear, think and do alike. Not only that but the question of self-identity of the individual clones wiI arise which may, perhaps, lead to abnormally abuse of individual freedom and identity of the clone persons also.

(c) The use of a clone, by the person of which it belongs, as means to his ends, can also not be denied. C. Claudia, a super model of Germany wishes to have two clones of her own to use them for getting herself free from her own burden of meeting to her numerous aspirant. Will it not be against the identity and freedom of an individual and, hence, immoral to use the human clones as one's means?

(d) Clone-technology is not sure on the subject of the mutation like forming of tumour and other unknown diseases that may unusually be caused by the artificial killing of the excess of *Y* chromosomes during processing of clones.

Asexuality and Lack of Emotional Attachment

(a) Clone is a creation out of asexual process. If animality is utterly neglected from the human person as in the cases of clones, there will be no possibility of proper imagination that arise in the midst of fascination, passion, emotion and other sublime human qualities. In lack of these human qualities, there will not only be the question of isolation and danger of deformation of the clone person but of survival also.

(b) If the person of which the clone is prepared, is an under aged, there may be a risk of not getting maturity of mind till death and if it belongs to a person of overaged there is all risks of getting elderly soon as we find in the case of Dolly.

(c) Not only that but there will be the problem of relation of the person with his clone because of the reason that the stem cell will be prepared from the same genetic source and, thus, the relation of the persons with their clones in respective cases will be of brothers/sisters and not of father/ mother and, thus, there will be cases of identity of relation and possibility of dehumanization.

(d) The clone person, I am not sure on the issue, is, perhaps, a being of a asexual category. In that case he/she will be of a non-sexual temperament and isolated from emotional attachment. He/she may get depressed in the absence of these human qualities, which are causes of attraction that makes life worth living. In his attachmentless life he may think of his life incomplete, purposeless and isolated and that may lead him to self-suicidal.

Deformation of Family

(a) No family is possible without marriage and no genius person will like to enter into family by marrying a wife of different level of brilliance as he may think of uncertainty of the quality of the offspring to be born out of their conjugal relation. Rather he/she will prefer to a get an identical clone of his/her own and thus, there will be a case of deformation not only of the family but of the whole hereditary system also.

(b) Who will be called the mother of the clone baby? The problem of real and surrogate mother will arise.

(c) In the cloning system women will be privileged because they are genetically fit self-creators if it is so, there is no need of men for the birth of a clone baby but similar is not the case in *vice versa* as man's cloning requires egg that cannot be possible without a woman. There will be no need of a male member in the family and, thus, there will be the cases of rise in the disproportionate population of female and desertion of males and thus, imbalance not only in the proportion of the two but in the nature itself also.

4. Division and Moral Deformation of Society

(a) The society will, then, obviously be divided in two categories of the clone class and of the lower class. The former will be a category of highly genius supermen while the latter of deprives. The former will occupy all high positions, services of high ranks and power and the latter will be unable to compete them. Deprived category of persons, for their survival, may get perversion and may cause violence in the society. The clones will not mix with the rest on the ground of the principle of inequality and the rest will be deprived and disregarded.

(b) The morality in society will also be divided into the

morality of the clones and that of the rest that is, herd or utilitarian morality. The clones, like Friedrich Nietzsche's superman, may claim that the utmost duty of the society is to rear clones who only have the right to live on earth. The morality of the clones based on the idea that 'all that proceeds from the power is good and all that springs from weakness is bad' will upset the moral aim of equality and peace in the society.

(c) As the cloning of man inevitably requires women's egg, of which the nucleus is taken out, there will be a dependency on women but in the *vice versa* there is no requirement of sperm; the very presence of men will be needless and, therefore, existence of men will be questioned that would lead to disorder in the society.

(d) The uniqueness and diversity of the qualities of human person in the society will be affected very badly as there will be a flood of the clones having uniformed qualities.

(e) A person may have a number of his clones at a time and, thus, it will be an unwanted and very dangerous cause of high rising population. Not only that but if the cloning, as industry is established, there will be cases of hiring wombs and that will not only be immoral but irreligious also.

(f) The number of orphan children will not only be rapidly raised high but there will be no solution to the problem of orphan adaptation also because the orphan-adapters of today would like to have a clone of their own rather than to adapt an orphan.

Deformation of Democracy

Insisting on trans-valuation of the values the clones or supra - rational will distinguish themselves from the herd with an unbridgeable difference and inequality. In that case equality will be a synonym of weakness, a moral standard for the herd or mediocre, who have no right to live in the kingdom of ends, while inequality will be natural in the eyes of the clones. We know that equality is the basis of democracy and, thus, the acceptance of inequality as natural will disintegrate the democratic pattern and behaviour.

Killing of Embryos

In the process of cloning a number of embryos has to be slayed, which is not only an immoral act but is irreligious sin also.

On the basis of the aforementioned disadvantages it is said by opponents that any technology, and hence, cloning, if there is possibility of causing wreckage, to a modern society of consumer by it, can't be pushed to flourish on the name of technological advancement.

Substitute

According to the recent technological inventions the excess of *Y* chromosome in the embryo, in mother's womb, destroys chromosomes bearing superman qualities and promotes the chromosomes causing perversion. Modern technology has invented such rays that can effectively destroy the excess of *Y*, in the womb of the mother herself, and this confers favour in promoting chromosomes bearing supermen qualities. On account of this process a woman longing for birth of a child endowed with superman qualities can get relief that she would have not to suffer the life of severe sanctimoniousness and austerity for more than nine months as prescribed by Indian scriptures.

In order to insure that supermen qualities can only develop and the inhuman and the anti-human qualities cannot, the Indian scriptures have prescribed some disciplines regarding the *sattvika* meal and healthy thoughts promoting *sattva* in parents before their intercourse with a desire to have such a child and after the fertilization as well. They prescribe certain norms for controlling sexual and other senses and concentration for sublimation of thoughts, their daily routine of eating, drinking, thinking and doing during pregnancy for the flow of *sattva*, the baby in mother's womb in a natural way. This flow of *soma* is effective in balancing the qualities 23-23 and, thus, making them stronger than Y chromosomes bearing deforming qualities and, consequently, leads not only to a total implantation of chromosomes bearing virtuous qualities but also in making them stronger than those of opposites, on account of which the advent of supermen as evidenced by scriptures, is made possible.

Gunasutras 23-23, in number, combined in embryo, may be such that :

1. The number of chromosomes bearing superman qualities is more than those bearing infra qualities which cause the birth of supermen.
2. The number of chromosomes bearing infra-qualities is more than these bearing superman qualities, which cause the birth of an individual of perverted or deformed nature.
3. Chromosomes bearing supermen qualities are stronger than those bearing infra qualities, which cause the birth of an individual of excellent qualities.
4. Chromosomes bearing infra qualities are stronger than those bearing supermen qualities, which cause the birth of a deformed person.
5. In cases when the number and strength of chromosomes bearing those separate qualities are, approximately equal, there is possibility of an ordinary individual.

Clone baby, as I know (and I very quickly add that I do not know it) will be different from all of those possibilities. If I create my Clone, my good qualities will be restored in it but the good qualities of my wife will not. But if the excellent qualities of both of the mother and the father are restored, as it occurs in some cases of heredity, and then if by technology we destroy the negative qualities of the parents in the embryo, there is possibility of creation even of super super- man and even so without disturbing the genetic system. In this way it is ethically neither needed nor preferable to change in heredity and social structure, based on it, by human cloning and with the help of technology a baby in a genetically manner, without cloning, may be created by destroying the bad qualities, highly unwanted, of the parents in embryo itself. Different from it, if all negative qualities of a person are destroyed, as it is done in cloning the person will not be different from a machine. There is every possibility of alteration and other typical diseases in clones also.

Conclusion

It can be said safely, as we have discussed earlier, that bioethical values can well be preserved and supermen can be produced even in genetic system by applying the biotechnology of destroying bearing qualities, highly unwanted, and promoting the chromosomes bearing excellence in embryo in the mother's womb. Promoting Sattva by adopting proper disciplines and sublimating thoughts, for making the chromosomes, bearing excellence, more dominant, is natural and non-risky. This way, there will be no fear of losing identity and freedom of a clone different from the person of which it is a cloned, of deformation of the human nature and of moral and as observed earlier, based on hereditary system.

I may be charged of being conservative of a type, who opposes all steps for novelty and progress in the beginning, with a fear of a risk against traditional order and values. One may also say that it is foolishness to criticize a move not materialized so far. It is reasonable to say let the human clone be created, then observe its excellence and behaviour and then evaluate it. If, otherwise, it will be only a guess work and, hence, unsteady. These all charges don't belong my views in the paper if I clarify that my analysis, in the paper, is the analysis of the concept formed in my mind by informations I acquired from different sources. However, I don't think that other will agree with my views in full but one can't deny the labour I have taken in exposing the ethical issues of human cloning.

Before conclusion the discussion, in this chapter, I think it is obligatory on my part to consider the ethics of biotechnology and the morality of the Biotechnologicians and Bioengineers involved in cloning. It cannot be a devil's task because they are also men of our society and, hence, cultured and knowledgeable persons in the world. While indicating to the nature, field, scope and aim of the bioethics, I, in the beginning of my talk, have already told that the morality of the biotechnologicians and engineers is to preserve any excellence and to manifest the human reason and power, assigned to them, to its highest extent and, thus, estimating from this point of view, their task of cloning cannot be termed immoral. Human cloning is not against the religious faith that God is the only creator because I find a basic difference between the creations by God, as some of the religions accepted, and the human cloning by the bio-scientists. Those religions themselves accept that God creates everything out of nothing but in human cloning bio-technologicians and engineers create clones not out of nothing but out of the genetic material to be precise, cells of the human body. Not only that but those religions may not deny that the power and excellence of the biotechnologicians and engineers are also assigned naturally to them by God and they are ordained to manifest them to the highest extent.

Chapter 8

Ageing : A New Look

M.P. Chourasia

Ageing is an age-old problem of human civilization. Since time immemorial, thinkers have advanced their views on the topic concerned. In Ayurveda certain medicines and valuable diets have been searched out to postpone ageing and to enhance longevity. At that time, people were not aware of the fact that the longevity of our life were corollary of physical factors. Even today there are many people who do not know the importance cf physical factors to postpone the ageing. They think that the length and breadth of human life depend on the mercy of God. *Ṛgveda* is full of such prayers,

पश्येम शरदः शतं जीवेम शरदः शतम्।
श्रृणुयाम शरदः शतं प्रबवाम शरदः शतम्।
अदीनाश्याम शरदः शतं भूयश्च शरदः शतम्।। ऋग्वेद

In other words, even those days people were eager to enjoy life of hundred years with healthy ears and vision. They prayed God to provide them many sons and cows to enjoy the earthly pleasure.

But in those days, science was not so developed to find out the cause of ageing. Human life is not fully physical. Human life does not fully depend on body, rather to some extent, it depends on inward conditions also. It is partly physical and partly spiritual. So life has two aspects: physical and spiritual or mental. The problem of ageing is closely related with body, not with life. Wrongly people have conceived that with the decay or end of the body life also ends. One who knows the real nature of life knows that he does never die. Old age and death are the physical phenomenon and it is body that vanishes. Why body becomes old? Because it is limited by world and governed by nature. Body is vehicle upon which human life travels. Why and how body is vehicle? Because it is congregation of thirteen organs that bear human life. Those are : Eyes, ears, nose, teeth, tongue, hands, mouth, legs, genital, anus, nostrils, nerves and mind. These organs together are friends of human life and also the foes. As long as these organs are working well, we are called healthy. But a time comes when these organs do not function in proper manner. Or their functioning are decreasing day-by-day. Human life comes from the unknown, and as long as it follows nature and maintains its character, it cannot be limited by the world. So life in a body is always related to its organs (*Taopanishad*-50-51). Human life fully depend on environment, because constitutive systems of life are always governed by environment. In one sense longevity of human life is a multiplication of environment and traits of body.

So to enhance the longevity or to postpone ageing, human being needs to improve the environment and body. Medical science conceives that if food conditions are balanced body will remain maintained and it will help us to increase the human longevity. We have six sources of balanced foods, those are: vitamins, minerals, proteins, carbohydrate, fats and water. If every element of these food factors are fulfilled in a balanced way, the human life will enjoy its full length. If one of these elements run short, it will hamper the human age. So to increase the longevity of human life, we have to maintain the food conditions. Human beings need intake of proper vitamins, minerals, proteins, fats, carbohydrate and hormones to enhance and stay ageing.

But this is partial truth. Only maintenance of food conditions are not enough to enhance the longevity of human life. For this purpose maintenance of internal and external organs of the body is necessary preconditions. In this regard physical labour, exercise or *yoga* is also necessary. By the former source, one can easily maintain one's body fitness while the latter, i.e., give physical *yoga* is able to mental and moral fitness. For the longevity of life to be tension free is necessary. One important cause of aging is mental tension because it creates hypertension. Hypertension further creates diabetes and other diseases which not only causes ageing but even untimely death. The root of all tensions is endless human desires and ambitions. If our desires are properly regulated, they will never create tension in life. Desire can be restrained with the help of *dhyan* and *yoga*. The practice of some moral virtues are preconditions of controlling the desires. According to Patanjali *Satya*, *ahimsa*, *asteya*, *aparigraha* and *brahmacharya* are those virtues that help individuals to diminish his desire. If we have no desire to harm others there will be no tension. If we have no wrong desire to deprive other person's thing in an immoral way, there will be no tension? So, the first step of mental purification starts with following of moral path and *yoga* and *dhyana*.

The *yoga* not only helps individual to maintain mental fitness but also physical fitness. In *pranayam*, individual inhale excess oxygen than what is essential in a *yoga* position. The excess inhaled oxygen nourishes the cells of those organs that are the centre of *yoga* position. For example, in *Padmasan* the circulation of blood is confined within the central part of the body more than in the legs. So is the case with *halasan* and *sarvangasan*. These *asanas* with *pranayam*, supply proper oxygens to the cells of brain, lungs and heart to maintain their capacity to work smoothly. If heart, lungs and brain work properly the other organs of the body will also function well. These together help to increase the longevity of individual's life. Our society also like those people's longevity who are self dependent and avoid those who are not. Because persons who are dependent are burdens for the society.

Recent development is genetic engineering considers gene defect as an essential factor of *aging* have already discussed the importance of *yoga* and *pranayam* in fighting against ageing and in maintenance of body's cells. If body's cells are properly maintained, they will be capable enough to fight against diseases and by doing so, they can protect the body for a long period. But weak cells are unable to fight against the diseases and are caught by fatal diseases. And in this way people either die soon or lose their health. According to the genetic engineering, if healthy gene is selected from chromosome and fertilized with healthy ovum in a laboratory, male/female so born could be able to fight against ageing and thereby increase longevity. According to this Genetic Engineering man/woman sexual conjugations, marriages and love are meaningless in producing a child. The whole authority of creation will be genetic engineer, who will control the creation with the help of computer. God will not be needed further more. In future, genetic engineering may search out those electro-magnetic and molecular factors of the human body that can change the construction of mind and the way of thinking. Consequently with the help of genetic engineering we can produce tension free man/woman. And such deed will enhance the longevity of human life.

But mere genetic engineering is not the sole factor. Longevity of man also depends on the local environmental factors. So even genetically produced child also requires suitable environment.

Today, we are living in a polluted environment in which the percentage of carbon dioxide and carbon monoxide are increasing day-by-day. Deforestation is making the land barren. Pesticide and other chemicals are poisoning the soil day-by-day. There are many industries and factories that flow their refuse in the holy rivers. Consequently, rivers of India are suffering from water pollution today. Our physical and bio-environments have been completely polluted. So, it is impossible to get pure water to drink and fresh air to breathe. In this situation to increase the longevity of human life is next to impossible. Because impurity of environment is one of the factors of ageing. So, if we want to enhance life-span, we must have to improve our environment first. Human life is the product of environment and food systems. Only the improvement of food standard is not sufficient to enhance the human longevity.

In recent period many scientists have emphasised the theory

of *natural selection*. This theory is based on the observation that the force of natural selection on survival in higher animals drops after the earliest age of reproduction is reached. As per this theory, ageing have evolved because genes that produce deleterious effects late in life meet little or no opposition from natural selection and thus become rampant in the gene pool. If this is to be believed, then progressively retarding the declining strength of natural selection for a number of generations in a test population should lead to the evolution of significantly postponed ageing in that lineage. This has indeed been shown to be true in fruit flies of the genus *Drosophila* that have had reproduction delayed across 10 or more generations. Such a practice resulted in generation of fruit flies that lived two or three times longer than normal. Though the experiment with fruit flies has encouraged scientists to evolve strategies for implementing similar delays in humans, a big deterrent would be the fact that the results would be too slow to emerge. In practice, no immediate change would be observed in successive generations and a time period extending over several centuries will be needed to yield a significant increase in life span.

In terms of biochemical causes, it is increasingly being realised that hundreds of genetically determined biochemical pathways, involving cascades of molecular interactions, influence longevity. These can possibly be manipulated to postpone ageing. Anti-ageing studies in recent past have identified 'telomerase' as a potential therapy. Telomerase is an enzyme that acts on structures called telomers, which cuts the ends of chromosomes. Telomers shrink a bit every time a cell divides when the length drops below a set threshold, cells stop dividing. Keeping this in view, it has been suggested that drug therapies that preserve telomers might enable dividing cells to reproduce and remain healthy for a long period. It has been proposed that such preservation might actually retard ageing of whole organism. This has, however, not been proved so far till date. A big caution that would always hinder such approach is that immortality of cells runs a great risk of promoting cancer. Additionally, a few genes have been identified in lower forms of life that could be involved in ageing process. Also, genetic analysis of long living humans has revealed existence of certain variable genes. It is still quite immature to conclude that these genes participate in postponing ageing, primarily due to the reasons that in all such studies sample size is too small and nothing much is known about the biological functions and unique features of the corresponding proteins. It might take a few more years by the scientists to ascertain this task through studies in the field of 'functional genomics'. Thus, it appears that alteration of the multifunctional ageing process is likely to require manipulation of several, perhaps many biochemical pathways.

With the recent developments in almost all branches of science, it seems plausible that the process of ageing might not be elusive for long. However, an immediate question that accompanies this optimum concerns of the end of such studies. Going by the basic human nature, there seems to be no limit to how long man's life can be extended. On the lighter side, there appears to be a few ethical and social problems waiting, in case of any success in this regard. Though such a scenario can only be speculated at this time, the postponement of human ageing would definitely raise difficult issues for public policy and personal ethics. Social securities and retirement age are just a few of them that come immediately to mind, apart from the potentially hazardous problem of overpopulation. In all, it would thus appear the serious problems that might arise as a result. A solution to the phenomenon of ageing is sure to bring with it tougher problems.

Considering the pros and cons arguments of science and bioethics we can say that even today science is in process of searching and what it has been searched out is not free from defects. From this point of view the solution forwarded by *yoga* is the best, because it follows the natural process through which one can develop resistance power of the body to fight against ageing in a natural way. And by this process the problem of over population can also be controlled with the help of self confinement.

Chapter 9

Ageing : A Psycho-Physiological Study— A Search from Cause to Cure

Shiva Nath Prasad

There is a popular proverb, "What cannot be cured must be endured". This proverb fits well for old age or for ageing. Ageing being a natural process, it is bound to occur to everyone, no one can help it. It compares well as an incurable disease, a worst disease, no one can help. It is beyond human control. The old age presents a pitiable spectacle, which moved Buddha to go for *tapas*, for an eternal remedy. At best one can try to adopt such an attitude in advancing years which may be called 'a sportsman spirit' and not take the advanced age as curse, or throw blame on any one, accept old age as inevitable stage, do not blame others for any sort of suffering, but remain mentally stable and calm and let life to flow in its natural way, like the stream which does not throw any blame for the ups and downs through which it has to traverse an uphill task, does not feel shattered or taken aback at the rise and fall through trials travails and tribulation. It is in the interest of enjoying life in every manner, that one should enjoy, all childhood, youth and also old age. This sort of attitude would change the very pattern of life, it would make life juicy, spicy and salty. Let life be a palatable dish of sweet and sour, hot and cold, ginger and onion. "If spring be, winter is left behind" or *vice versa*. The multiple morbidities of old age may not deter him (man) to miss the joys of youth. Let nature go its own course. In this background, we may enter into an academic discussion on old age or the ageing problem in its multi faced aspects.

Lord Mahabir's "*Saptabhangi*" presents a unique philosophy of relativism, which makes allowance for looking into things from several standpoints, and that every standpoint is right in its own way, without opposing the other. Similarly, if we want to explain the problem of ageing, we can see it in its various aspects. It cannot be summarily said at the very outset, if ageing is only a moral problem at all or it is essentially a social problem, or it is a legal problem, or it is a biological or physiological problem, a medical problem, or it is a psychological problem. These are some of the standpoints for looking at the problem of ageing. A coordinated approach which covers all the above is nearly the real approach. The basic fact is that it is a biological, or bio-chemical phenomena, which includes, what are known as the physiological-biological or biochemical phenomena that lead any one to become old? How does one know that a certain man is an old man? What are the signs of old age or ageing, why ageing? How should one avoid or delay the process of ageing? If one becomes old, what is the remedy to conquer it once for all? What are the adequate medicines which can cure old age or the ageing problem? These are some of the problems involving old age. Besides, there are other allied questions too, how should we behave with old man, what should we do for the satisfaction of the old man? What assistance should we offer to the old man, when he is really physically unable to play active part in the game of life? Should we adopt an attitude of reverence, or should we shun him for his financial or physical disability to his own offspring? These problems are related to socioethics. Scholars have tried to look into different ways, and in this chapter, I shall try to dwell upon on one aspect only and leave the rest problems for future occasions.

Whether ageing is a social problem, an ethical problem, a medical problem, economic problem, a philosophical problem, a psychological problem is a question of debate. But above all, it cannot be denied by anyone, whether he is a scientist, or philosopher, a political thinker, a social activist or a medical scientist, that enduring economic and social order of any nation-state can only be built on the solid foundation of justice, peace equality, security and liberty, whereby one can live in peace and ease without fear, eliminating all causes of insecurity, economic instability like poverty, illiteracy, inequality, unemployment, dependence, squalor or what Sir William Beveridge called "Freedom of wants", the Five Giants in the path of social progress — Want, Disease, Ignorance, Squalor, Idleness. It has been said by one scholar, that one of the most important social rights "Freedom from want" is most significant, and Dr. C.B. Memoria says, "As atom bomb is the most effective weapon of war, social security is the most effective weapon of peace". According to him, social security is the bedrock of all economic plans, it is one of human rights of people to get protection against social risks, it is a recognition of inherent dignity and equal fundamental rights of all members of human family, it is the foundation of freedom, justice and peace and of the equality. The International Labour Organisation Report of 1942 included under this social security, speaks to cover risks like sickness, maternity, invalidity, old age and death. The I.L.O. says that there are two stages of dependence in the life of everyone, *firstly* childhood, and *secondly* old age. It is bound by the canons of security of the parents to support a child in childhood, as it is a helpless stage, and the child to support the parents in old age. As early as 1883, the Chancellor of Germany Bismarck, included under the ambit of social insurance, sickness, *old age* and infirmity. A committee of Economic Security constituted President Roosevelt in 1834, provided for security against two great disturbing factors of life, which included unemployment and *old age*. In America in 1943, the Wagner-Murray Dingall Bill was introduced, which provided relief for "General welfare," to alleviate the economic hazards *of old age*, premature death, disability, sickness, unemployment and dependency. In 1934, Prof Adarkar had pleaded for scheme *for old age pension.* The problem of old age has been included under social assistance and social insurance. The invalidity and *Old Age Convention* 1933, provides for the granting of non-contributory allowances, *as of right to the needy invalids and old persons*. Non-contributory old age pensions have been provided in New Zealand (1898), Australia (1901-08), France (1919), Norway (1923), South Africa (1928). The U.S. Social Security Act 1935 encouraged for *old age pensions*. These facts show that the problem of old age is a recurrent problem and in its solution, ethical considerations are no less involved, i.e., the basic tenets of morality being rightness and wrongness of human conduct, liberty, justice, peace, security, etc., then the political, social, economic or even the psychological problems. If these are met, where has one to go to search for ethics?

Now, what is old age? It is very difficult to define old age. Different persons give different definitions based on their emphasis on their own choice of interests. To politicians and industrialists, it means power and wealth, whereas to a middle class employer, it means forced retirement, for the poor, it is a state of complete dependence on others; and for a woman, it is a loss to her charm and attraction; for the economists, it has reference to a poverty laden state and instable economic condition; for a politician, it indicates political insecurity, lack of justice, equality, loss of individual rights, for the social scientist, it indicates social disparity and discrimination; for a moral thinker, it refers to the human sentiments guided by mutual trust, respect, obedience of duty, keeping care to *the old man's* desires, want, and convenience, to medical scientist, it is a biological problem, for going down of health, requiring proper treatment, it is for a modern man more a subject of Biotechnology, Biochemistry, Gerontology and the science of Geriatrics, as such *study of old age* or ageing requires a multi-disciplinary approach.

There are group of scholars, who have divided the problem of old age or ageing into three groups, (i) socio-cultural, and in this very group, they also include the emotional and psychological aspects, (ii) the economic aspect, and (iii) health and medical care problems. The first group is the most important and it covers such a wide range of aspects of *old age* that this aspect needs too much to be said, it is a subject of a full and independent paper, including psychological, sociological, cultural aspects. Something can be said in this regard in a nutshell. In the psychological sense, old age is the most unrelished, deprived, discarded and alienated stage of life. It is really an alienated stage not only from others but from his own self. In old age, when he has to live a very deprived life, all the members of the family try to avoid him, he is no longer consulted in any matter, even he craves for a company, no younger person likes to sit before him and use a consoling, comforting word for him. Even food is served to him, but not with respect, but it is, as if, is to be given to the servants or thrown before the dogs; only some remnants of food taken by other members of the family is given to him. His frail body does not allow him to care for his own body, his extreme dependence leads him to wait for the other members of the family to give some relief, as if a drop of ambrosia in the mouth of that man. The old man who was one day in the hub of family life, is now a rejected lot, a rotten thing, fit for the dustbin and the younger persons waiting for his death, waiting sooner than ever. While the old man relishes to call or invite his friends and relative, his married daughters, etc., for sweet words of consolation or for a recreation, the younger people don't like that anyone should come to see him. They feel humiliation. The non-owners of any sort of property, or a pensioner, are most deprived lot. The psychological depression on this account leads him either to be forced to think that he is an *unwanted, valueless figure* or sooner he dies the better. This feeling reduces his life span. This is most cruel stage of affairs.

In this regard, as it has been said above, old age is a multi-faced alienation and needs to be mentioned here how alienation is very important factor of old age.

Alienation : Alienation may be defined for the purpose of ageing, as a state of powerlessness, normlessness, isolation and meaninglessness. Powerlessness is a stage or means or refers to a stage, which makes the individual feel that he has no authority or say in any of the matters. Normlessness creates the feeling that the social roles, standards or values are no more observed. Isolation is a stage where the individual happens to feel that he is all alone and there is none who came to his aid and listen to him. Meaninglessness is a stage where the individual feels that his existence is of no use and he has no utilitarian value for society.

Researches reveal that growing age was of no consequences, rather state of health was more important, man suffering from poor health had a greater feeling of meaninglessness and powerlessness. Feeling of powerlessness, normlessness was predominant on non-functioning aged persons than functioning ageds; non-effective heads had more of such feeling of powerlessness, normlessness than effective heads. Economic dependence is also important in these. The widowers most suffer from feeling of isolation and meaninglessness. Psychological experiments reveal that the widower's life span get reduced after the death of the wife, while that of widows, their life span increases in view of the fact that after she/they become widow, they have to fight with problems of life to maintain her/their children, which required more courage, toil, the will to live. But just opposite is the case with the widower. They become fed up with the problems of life due to strain in looking after their children, etc.

The uneducated men are found to be more dictatorial and they suffer from all the above defects. The old men who were not in service previously, suffer more from normlessness, powerlessness and isolation than their counterparts, as they believed in the conventional authority of the elderly people. If the possessions of the old persons are not transferred to their children, these defects may be reduced. If the widowers are provided with the company of their compeers, preferably of opposite sex such feeling gets minimized. The old persons should also try to leave their dictatorial role. Solution can be found also by providing "Senior Citizens" Homes, where they are assured of work, food, clothing, shelter, liberty, care, good medical aid, and above all company.

The psychological problem of personal alienation may be due to several factors. (i) Sudden change from occupational engagement to occupational retirement, and then apart from economic consequences of withdrawal from active life, i.e., depression, loneliness, frustration, unhappiness; forced retirement is no less than cancer (ii) death of close friends, relatives, involve loneliness; and (iii) longevity involves living in social, economic and value systems. One more factor which creates adverse effects in the minds of the elders, is the fear of becoming old or fear of death. Acute feeling in this regard, tells heavily on the psyche of the aged person.

Care of the aged involves several problems and for this, a very comprehensive programme requires to be chalked out, with the help and co-operation of the psychologists, social reformers, social scientists, economists, medical scientists, so that overall life of depression, loneliness of the aged be avoided and the feeling of "being aged or old" does not come in the mind of the aged, which is a great depressing factor.

Tuckman and Large in his studies found that *old* person become stubborn, touchy, engaging in quarrels with their children and always try to remain bossy, meddling with other people's affairs. Golde and Koyen in their studies found that younger people have negative perception of the old. Becker and Taylor expressed mixed views. They found that students living with grand parents endorse fewer negative stereotypes about the aged than those living with parents only. The young person finds in old person "prying into affairs of others" but these can be remedied by proper education. Young persons dislike old persons because of their untidy living, unclean living, living a shabby life, keep the room in which they live in uncleaned condition, keeping everything in haphazard way, topsy-turvy way. Further, the young people dislike the presence of old person because they feel that the old man expect all others to like him, honour him, respect him, do everything he likes or says. This gives rise to a feeling of discomfort and disliking of the young towards the old persons. This can also be remedied by proper education. The young people fail to realise that one who is young today will also become old some day. If they understand the factor of "generation gap", lacking understanding between the young and old, communication and appreciation of the behavioural patterns, values, mannerisms between young and old, much of the dislikes of the young would be reduced. The younger generation suffer from the lack of understanding with regard to the feeling of the old and the aged. They fail to realise that old age marks a shift in individual's position from active social participation to a state of marked decline in role-playing and performance and from economic self-sufficiency to economic dependence. Such types of changes result in a change of behaviour and habits of the elderly which sometimes irritate the younger ones. The negative attitude of younger generation towards the aged and elders can be changed by increasing their level of consciousness in the family, their changing status and reformulate their social and psychological roles. The younger ones need to be sensitised to understand the need and problems of the elders, with greater sympathy and tolerance. The greatest difficulty with the youth is that, the youth oriented society tries to dislocate the aged and in psychological terms, the old are forced to *feel old*, they become 'aged' because they are forced to feel aged and counting days for death. This psychological ailment does havoc and life of the aged becomes doomed.

A majority of scholars stress that cultural factors have important bearing in the process of ageing. Scholars for a long period, considered diversity of cultural configuration having its impact on ageing and investigated cross-cultural images and attitudes, first, by ethnographically examining a wide variety of cultural contexts, regularities and patterns as regards treatment of older individuals and seemed, by assessing the effects of major cultural changes upon how the elderly are integrated and treated in their respective culture. Anthropologists who see age in a cultural domain accept it as denoting the progression of individuals through major divisions of life cycle and argue that all cultures must resolve the questing of structuring age differences.

American scholars have greatly emphasized the psychological aspect of ageing. Several cinema shows are organised in America for this purpose. They stressed a development of personality complex of an individual and bearing of socio-cultural variable upon it. Differences in adjustment was examined by working out the extent of interaction between psychological variable, in the socio-cultural matrix of the American society. *Five adaptative* tasks for the aged were identified: recognition of ageing, and definition of instrumental limitations, redefinition of physical and social life space, substitution of alternative sources of need satisfaction, reassessment of criteria for evaluation of the self and reintegration of value, and life goals. This approach is the reminder of the fact that ageing is purely a mental process and to view it purely by physiological approach is to ignore personality configuration of an individual. It is agreed that decline in mental capabilities does *not entail corresponding change in physiology; rather decline in physical health precedes decline in mental health.*

Thus we have seen vast importance of psychological, socio-cultural, emotional factors in the process of ageing as well as the fallout of ageing. But how is it that the physiological factor is most important, it is only the medical scientists, the doctors, the geriatric scientists, the gerontologists can say and also say how far can the medical science go to remedy ageing, delay ageing, or cure ageing. Jeff Beaubier has acutely examined on the biological facts responsible for ageing. According to him, "Ageing is an increasing interference in the randomness in the biological organisation". Two directions of research are discernible first, is an attempt to look for specific genes which initiate ageing; others identify increased randomness in biological molecules as the cause of ageing. Some other opine that ageing consisted of two simultaneous components, anabolic building up and catabolic breaking down.

Further two types of approaches to ageing problems were also in use, endogenous and exogenous. Endogenous line of thinking recognises the diminished role of cellular functions whereas exogenous line of thinking presuppose, ageing to be associated with pathological processes. In the long run, this process combines to bring about the end of individual. It is also stressed that during the early years, the process of ageing is not rapid and this phase of men's life is called senescence. This phase is succeeded by the phase of rapid decline in one's cognitive thinking. This stage is characterized by senility. For the reason that old age is unavoidable, more attention should be given to healthy living of old age than to increase the life span.

There are scholars according to whom genetic factors play important role in the process of ageing, but they also opine that environmental factors can alter the cause of the process drastically. There are many theories explaining the ageing process. Rate of living theory postulates that there is only a limited amount of vitality and that the individual can choose to use it up quickly and live short life or slowly live a long one. This is very much like the wear and tear or stress theory of ageing.

There is one Collagen theory which postulates that with the time of the collagen of the body, which makes up large fraction of body protein, becomes more and more rigid and interferes with normal organ function.

There is another theory about ageing known as *Auto-immune theory.* This postulates, that change (perhaps a mutation) occurs in some of the cells of the immune recognition system in such a way that they do not recognise certain somatic cells as belonging to individual. An immune reaction takes place which leads to various auto-immune diseases.

There is *Somatic mutation theory* which states that spontaneous mutation occurs in the somatic cells causing them and their progeny to perform a different function from that performed in the original tissue. This theory is usually acceptable. Any hastenable change in a cell is considered a mutation. This could include gene mutations, chromosome aberrations or even de-differentiation. All somatic cells undergo spontaneous mutation, and once a cell has suffered a mutation, it may lead to degenerative diseases. The reason why a man lives so much longer than a mouse, for example, is because his spontaneous mutation rate is very much lower. The science of Biotechnology and Genetic Engineering give much detail and those who want to have detailed knowledge may consult those books together with books on Geriatrics-Gerontology.

Our medical science is in a fast developing stage and great medical scientists are trying to find out some such medicine which can increase man's life span, delay the ageing process and to bring old age in healthier position. Lack of medical care, poverty, mal-nutrition, unhealthy diet are also factors which lead to ageing, even prematurely. Many drugs have been put into investigation so that their use may retard ageing process one way or the other. One main consideration in the use of any drug is that the drug used should be free from side-effects. The medical scientists have found that one drug "Centrophenoxine" has attained the status of an "ageing-reversal" agent because of its various anti-ageing effects with almost no effects in clinical trials even after chronic administration. The short name of this drug is CPH. which works with chemical effect of lipofuscin which is considered to be irreversible. Besides the Cipfuscinolytic activities of CPH, the drug has presented many anti-ageing effects. CPH reduces water-insoluble protein content of the brain and living of the ageing experimentals, it increases the protein synthesis. No other substance has been proved more useful in the therapy of elderly and altering the age associated inevitable changes as CPH which thus can rightly be assigned the status of a true "Ageing-reversal" substance.

Regarding economic factors leading to old, state should really own the responsibility and all social measures may be adopted as laid down in the beginning of the chapter whereby social security measures have been discussed. Medical factors are essential and that aspect should be covered by the state, so that the aged and elderly have not to depend upon their younger who are unable or unwilling to invest out of their incomes.

One more factor which I wish to add in this connection but start with a question. What age should be taken to be proper age for keeping anyone in the category of the Old? The question relates to medical science, but the doctors are not really able to draw up a line or limit, to declare anyone in the category. Some countries, adopt age 60 as the year for being old, and accordingly in such countries old age pension starts after sixty. Some countries adopt 65 years, but generally 60+ is the guiding line. But this fact does not hold for all. There are persons who look aged much before they have come up to 60 years of age. There are also persons who look young and energetic even in much higher age. There are fools and knaves who behave like mentally retarded person, and age is no consideration. There are boys of small age, who behave much like an old man. Hence, age cannot be the only criteria for deciding anyone as aged or elderly. A better way of understanding would be that if a man is old or elderly, wisdom of age must peep into it, otherwise there would be no differences whether a man is 20-30 years or above 60. This question would lead to conceptual analysis of the problem of ageing, which would make a study, an understanding of aged/elderly, which would be interesting and informative study, really a philosophical study.

The cause of aged or elderly is a matter of great humanness, it is crucial since everyone has to pass through this stage, so everyone should be firm in mind to serve the cause of the aged, old and elderly. It is a great social cause to serve the older people with softness, tolerance, humanness and by so doing one can serve the nation also and bring peace and prosperity. Shakespeare through King Lear, perhaps epitomises and symbolises the sufferings of the old age-

Oh heavens,
"If you do love old men.....
"if you yourself are old,
Make it your cause...."

Let us all make it a cause and serve the needy, the depressed, the solitary, the alienated, the destitute, who need a healing touch, soft words, sweet behaviour.

In this twenty first century, the medical science have progressed immensely. Though as yet medical science has not succeeded in conquering death but at least, it has succeeded in prolonging life from 27 years average to seventy years, it has added years to life, the day would not be far off when life span in its most healthy state would go for full hundred years as we find, in our Indian *sastras "jivema sharadam sitah*, end life after one hundred years in the last *sannyas ashram* in the lap of nature, a wilful death away from hospitals, enjoy. *The World Health Organisation Bulletin*, in as early as 2001, in its declaration at Helsinki opined "Advances in medicine depends on innovative and bold clinical research, much of the progress we have seen in the effectiveness and safety of disease treatment, diagnosis and prevention is the result of intensive research involving human subjects. The research has undoubtedly been in the interests of health of individuals and general public, clinical research, however, must be ethically acceptable as well as scientifically sound. Ideally, every clinical study conducted anywhere in the world should respect the same internationally recognised clinical standards."

Besides the vast achievements of our medical scientists, the *yogic* methods of *pranayama* can also go a long way in healing multiple disease, making man healthy and also by *yogic sadhana* end life in meditative states away from the pains of death by way of completing a journey as it were.

Chapter 10

Ageing : Towards A More Technical Study — Biomedical Aspects

Shiva Nath Prasad

Definition

Ageing may be defined as the progressive deterioration in the structure and functions of the cells, tissues and organs of an organism with the advance age.

The average life span of different organism differ from individual to individual, some live only for small period, other live a life of several decades, but none can live forever and conquer death. After birth, one passes through the stages of growth, maturation and senescence phase and ultimately meets death. In common circumstance, the animals or any other creature live normal span of life except those who fall victim of any fatal accidents, disease, etc. Growth normally continues till 25 years. Thereafter many organs start showing gradual decline in their functional activities. Some of them may even regress in size. As an organism grows older, its power of metabolism gradually declines and its capacity to replace the worn-out cells and to repair the damage parts decreases. The cells, tissues and organs gradually become weak to perform the functions effectively. These changes result in the decreased adaptability of the animals to its environment. These changes appearing with advancing age are known as ageing. They occur in all organisms and ultimately lead to their death. During the phase of ageing cardiac output, filtration rate of kidney, homeostatic mechanism, etc., decreases. However, the decrease differs from organ to organ and also from individual to individual. The capacity of resistance to various diseases also becomes less efficient in old animals.

The life-span of different living organism can be understood in the following way—

Mayfly's life-span	-	*24 hrs.*
Silk moth	-	*2-3 days*
Rat	-	*4 years*
Rabbit	-	*13 years*
Monkey	-	*26 years*
Dog	-	*26-30 years*
Toad	-	*36 years*
Cat	-	*35-40 years*
Chimpanzee	-	*40 years*
Horse	-	*60 years*
Elephant	-	*65 years*
Man	-	*100 years*
Parrot	-	*140 years*
Tortoise	-	*200 years*
Sequoia	-	*3000-4000 years.*

Recent researches show that women's life-span is longer than men because the biological process of ageing is faster in human male than human female though apparently it does not seem so. Japanese have longest life span, i.e., 76.3 years in male and 82.5 years in female. Average life-span of an Indian is 59 years. However, in Kerala, male life expectancy is 69 years while that of female is 74 years.

Indian Ayurvedic science as well as *Yoga Sastra* of India point out that higher or long or short life-span of any organism depends upon the number of breathes per minute the particular organism or living being takes. The creatures which takes lesser number of breathes per minute stay longer than those creatures which more breathes per minute.

It may be mentioned here that the *Yoga Sastra* has devised a very comprehensive system of *pranayama*, which is also called 'breath control', *prana + ayam*, which literally means dimensions of *prana*, which (*pranayam*) by controlling breath and taking less breath per minute than the normal breath per minute, man can enlarge and enhance life-span at least for 100 years or even more. It is seen in general that when a man remains in healthy state, he takes normal breath, but when he become afflicted with disease, his breathing per minute increases. In acute cases of disease, heaving also starts rapidly. The English word 'disease' can be analysed as dis + ease, i.e., not in ease, or not comfortable or normal, but in Hindi or in Ayurvedic terms, man who is free from disease is called *swastha*, which word can be broken into two parts *swa + avasthita*, which means, placed within himself, in an inward directed *stage*. In Ayurvedic science, a healthy man is one whose *kaph*, *pitt* and *vayu* are all in equilibrium, when this equilibrium of three principles of life are broken, physical afflictions start. In *Samkhya* system, we find mention of *samyavastha* or equilibirum of *sattva*, *rajas* and *tamas*, with increase of one *guna* or quality or preponderance of one *guna* over other *guna*, lead to difference in the type, kind, quality of living of different individuals. If *sattva guna* prevails over *rajas* and *tamas*, the man is of *sattvik* kind, if *rajas guna* preponderates over the other two *gunas*, a man becomes *rajasik* type and when *tamas guna* preponderates over the rest two the man becomes of *tamasik* nature. The conception of '*Trimurti*' as Prof. S. Radhakrishnan says is a primitive concept coming from epic period and continues in the *Puranas*. This '*Trimurti*' can be translated in English as "Triad", i.e., three. *Prakriti* is a strand of three *gunas*. In its primeval state of *samyavastha*, there is no *sristi*, but when there is any disturbance in their position due to proximity of *purusa*, *sristi* starts. The *sattva guna* or equanimity, is born of wisdom, *rajas* or energy, is outcome of spirited feeling and *tamas* or heaviness, springs due to lack of enlightenment and control, these are the aspects of all existence, even God is not considered to be exception to it. There is a trinity of godhead. *Brahma*, *Visnu* and *Mahesh*, and *Brahma* is said to be *rajasi*, since He is the creator and as *rajas* is the principle of action, *Brahma* is called Rajasik.

Shiva as the principle of destroyer is said to be of *Tamasik* nature. *Prakriti* is the main cause of creation, it is uncaused (*aja*) one (*eka*) it is a strand of three *gunas* (*trigunatmika*) it has form (*sarupa*) since it creates the manifold. So it is called *Vahvi Praja*, it is *Pradhana, Avyakta* and *Sasvata* (eternal).

Samkhya is a metaphysical system, while *yoga* is a practical system. By the methods of *yoga*, which has eightfold steps, *yama, niyama, asana, pranayama, pratyahara, dharana, dhyan, samadhi.* The word *yoga* means to be unified and this being unified is *yoga*, united with Godhead. The various steps of the *yoga* are some of the ways to be united with Godhead or which is called *Ishwar Pranidhana. Yoga* is defined as *'chitta vṛiti nirodhah*, to control the meanderings of mind : *Pranayama* is the fourth step of *yoga*. This is connected with breath or *swasa* i.e., inhaling/exhaling. The process of taking breath (air) inside or in common language 'inhaling' is called *'swasa'*, while throwing out of breath air is called *praswasa* only when breath is retained, it leads to the fruition of *pranayama,* i.e., *pranayama sidhi.* With this is connected, the *ida nadi* and *pingala nadi* and the last is *susumna nadi*. By breath control one can captivate the serpant power *kundalini*. By the retention of breath or controlling of breath, one can enlarge one's life span, arrest ageing, arrest decrement of age-factors. Just as a tortoise takes few breaths in a minute, so it has a longer life than other beings, similarly by reducing the normal breathing rhythm, per minute, one can enlarge life-span. In the Himalayan jungles, even now there are *sadhus* wrapt in *yoga sadhana* for a long time and they have longer life than others and this life is a far healthy life than ordinary human beings. The secret of longer and healthy life lies in controlling breath *swasa praswasa* and so enjoy longer health. We have in the *Upanisad*, the story of the King Yayati, who took his youth from his son and enjoyed a long life with his wife for thousands of years. What does it mean? Life depends on breath. There are several medicines in Ayurveda science which lead to longer life, longer sexual vigour, enjoying several women, etc. In *Agni Purana* also, several such recipes have been given.

Though technically 'breathe' and *pranayama* are not identical but in common language both are taken to mean similarly. One fact is most important that, breathing is most essential for life and the moment, breath is stopped, one dies, this is the reason that in English there is an expression 'breathed his last' to mean death. When the breath is stopped finally, one dies. The air which we inhale or exhale is also called *Prana Vayu.* Without this *Prana Vayu,* no one can remain alive. The retention of *Prana Vayu* in the *Saharsrar* or in the *samadhi* state, the mental constructions stops, this stage is called *Param aham,* as distinguished from *Kshudra aham* or *bahya prapanch.* Technically *pranayama is not breath control but control of Prana and Prana Vayu. Prana* is also called the principle of activity or motion, including the cause of gravitation and magnetism. Dr. Umesh Kumar Sriwastawa in his paper on '*Pranayam*' (Published in Journal of *Bihar Philosophical Research* 2004) has quoted Swami Vivekananda explanation of the word *Prana* which is as follows, "It is *pranas* that is manifesting as the action of the body, as the nerve currents, as thought force down to the lowest force everything is but the manifestation of *prana.* The sum of all forces in the universe, mental or physical when resolved back to their original state is called *prana.* The knowledge and control of this *prana* is really what is meant by *pranayama. Prana* becomes Absolute Existence, attains omniscience, *Prana* is the vital force in everything including thought which is the highest and the finest of all actions. The action of *prana* is most suitable, in its finer state of vibration, the whole universe is composed of subtle vibration and all these are acts of *prana,* but this motion is not to be confused with breath, breath is not producing *prana,* on the contrary, but controlling that power which moved the lungs. The English translation of *breath* as *prana* is misleading, it is *prana* which is the basis of all actions, aspiration is also manifestation of *pranayam.* The mystical vision is also due to *prana.* Even the physical sciences are manifestation of *prana.* The control of *prana* as mental force is called *Raja Yoga*".

With this small description of *prana,* we can easily deduce that with these specialization and control of *prana/pranayam* miracles can be achieved, mystical vision can be attained and the stopping of ageing to a considerable extent is most possible. It requires more elaboration, how far can *pranayam* provide longevity, arrest ageing process, etc. and I shall devote one separate paper on "Ageing & Yoga" later. Medical science has yet to develop some method, or remedy for stopping ageing but this was very common with the Indian sages.

Signs of Ageing

The books on Gerontology, Giriatics, Biology and Bio-chemistry have suggested the signs of ageing which can be summed up as under different heads, and among those heads, two are most important :

(A) Morphological and Physiological

(i) The cells gradually lose the capacity retaining of water which leads to the decrease of blood volume, thus making the tissue drier.

(ii) Rapid coordination of body parts starting declining after thirty years of age.

(iii) Muscle tissue degenerates due to biochemical changes in the muscle fibres and neuromuscular functions. This leads to reduction of muscular strength.

(iv) The bones gain in mineral water and become brittle and more liable to fracture.

(v) Calcium accumulates in blood and other tissues.

(vi) Hair start greying or falling out after the age of 40 years.

(vii) Elasticity of ligaments between small bones in the back lessens after the age of 30.

(viii) Ability of the lungs to absorb and supply oxygen diminishes due to their decreased elasticity and increased rigidity of the chest wall. Less oxygen supply affects the working of heart, brain and muscles.

(ix) Heart muscle ages and this decreases cardio-vascular functions.

(x) Formation of new RBCs from the bone marrow slows down.

(xi) Cholesterol deposits on the inner surface of the arteries as a result of eating fatty food throughout life. This may block circulation or form blood clots that can disrupt vital functions of heart, brain and lungs.

(xii) Powers of hearing and sight progressively decrease from 30 and 50 years of age respectively. Hearing loss is often due to the wearing away of sensory hair in the inner ear as a result of repeated exposure over a long time to loud voice.

(xiii) Memory is slightly impaired at 60 years of age due to decrease in neurons. However, intellect remains quite sharp.

(xiv) Body may develop auto immunity, which the immune system turns against the body, attacking its cells as if they were invading organisms.

(xv) The body's immune system loses its ability to effectively deal with the antigens. This reduces resistance to infectious diseases.

(xvi) Thymus attains its maximum size shortly before sexual maturity and then gradually shrinks until it is almost microscopic by age of 70.

(xvii) Women stop menstruating at about 45-50 years of age.

(B) Cellular Changes

(i) Chromosomal abnormalities and gene mutations in the nuclei of the somatic cells cause changes in DNA structure. That disturbs the enzyme synthesis. For example, with the increase in age, the liver cells show more of chromosomal aberrations. The nucleus shrinks and strains deeply with advancing age. Thus condition is due to condensation of chromatin and leads to cellular death. Such a degenerative process is called *nuclear pyknosis*.

(ii) With the advancement of age in enzyme *aldolase* synthesized by the mice liver cells, becomes more and more inactive.

(iii) With increase in age, large quantities of *defective proteins* accumulate in the body cells. This is due to the increase in defects in the DNA.

(iv) DNA replication is retarded to a considerable extent.

(v) *Pigment accumulation* increases in the aged animals.

(vi) *Mitochondria* decrease and *lysosomes* increase in number.

(vii) *Endoplastric reticulation* decreases in old cells.

(viii) With advancing age bio-membranes are impregnated with calcium. This affects their biological role.

(ix) The lipids of bio-membranes of old cells break down forming a fatty, brown pigment *lipofucin*. The granules of this pigment accumulates in the muscles and nerve cells and interfere in their functioning.

(x) The size of nucleus decreases.

(xi) The body cells gradually lose the power of multiplication

(C) Intra Cellular Changes

(i) The body cells are surrounded by interstitial fluid, which contain several types of chemical compounds out of which *collagen proteins* is most abundant Collagen forms about 40 per cent of the protein contents of the body.

(ii) *Collagen* in young-age group is permeable, flexible and soluble, therefore, there is easy change of materials between the cell cytoplasm and interstitial fluid the rough semi-permeable membranes. But with advancing age, the *collagen* protein becomes less flexible, less permeable and insoluble. Due to these changes, there is a decreased in flow of nutritive substances and oxygen into the cells and also decrease loss of nitrogenous wastes and CO_2 in the body. This causes decreased efficiency of body cells and induces ageing in the cells and finally in the whole body.

Theories of Ageing— No area of biological inquiry is susceptible to such a large number of theories as in the science of gerontology, owing not only to the fact that there is sufficient lack of fundamental data but also because manifestations of biological changes with time affect almost all biological systems from molecular level upto the whole organism. It is, therefore, easy to construct a theory of ageing based on a biological decrement (or decline) that may be observed to occur in time in any system at the level of molecule, cell, tissue, organ or whole animal.

The question is : Is change observed a direct cause of ageing or is it the result of changes that may be occurring at a more fundamental level.

The Encyclopaedia of Bioethics says, "If the modern notions of biological developments are rooted in signals originating from information-containing molecules, then it would seem reasonable to attribute post-developmental changes to a similar system of signals occurring at the molecular level. One current theory of ageing rests on decrements occurring with time in the immune system such that individuals are less able to deal with infectious or antibodies "mistakenly" produced against their own cells. Either or both these events would lead to a reduced ability to deal with environmental insults, and thus an increasing force of mortality would result. That such events might occur cannot be wholly denied, but this logic would suggest that, conversely, "maturation" of the immune system in early life controls development of the animal. Conventional wisdom does not accept this as a likely possibility".

If age changes are caused by fundamental changes in information containing molecules that result in chain reaction fashion, in physiological decrements of higher organisational levels, that is, cell, tissue, organs whole animal then most tenable theories of ageing are those based on molecular events occurring in the genetic apparatus". (p. 48)

Several theories have been put forward on Ageing. in my previous paper, I have mentioned at least three theories. But here I wish to mention all the theories which are discussed in the Bio-technology and Bioinformatics :

(i) *Environmental Theory* — According to this theory, the adverse changes in the cellular environment cause ageing.

(ii) *Genetic Theory* — Some biologists believe that ageing in animals is dependent on an intrinsic genetic property of the cells of the body.

(iii) *Environmental-cum-Genetic Theory* — The process of ageing is an outcome of interaction between the genes and the environment. This theory includes both environmental theory as well as genetic theory.

(iv) *Collagen Theory* — It states that ageing is induced by changes in the collagen protein in the interstitial fluid surrounding the body cell.

(v) *Wear-and-Tear or Stress Theory* — It states that the cell and tissues of the body are always subjected to wear and tear processes due to changes in the intrinsic and extrinsic actors. These processes induce the symptoms of ageing in an individual, which finally dies.

(vi) *Metabolic Theory* — It states that those organisms which have higher metabolic rate, nature, age and die earlier than those organism which have low metabolic rate and take years to mature and years to age.

(vii) *Clinker's or Waste Product Theory* — It states that ageing is due to accumulation of metabolic wastes inside the body cells. These wastes beyond some limits, poison the body cells and decline the metabolic rate and induce ageing.

(viii) *Immunity Theory* — This theory suggests a link between ageing and disappearance of the thymus gland by late middle age in man. Thymus stimulates the proliferation of lymphocytes, increasing resistance of infection. Absence of this gland affects in two ways :

(a) It weakens the body's natural defence against foreign germs; and

(b) It increases the number of abnormal cells formed in the body itself. This destroys the tissues.

(ix) *Cross-Linkage Theory* — According to this theory, ageing is caused by increase in the bonds between protein and nuclei acid molecules in the all, thereby altering the functional characteristics of these important cellular compounds.

(x) *Error Catastrophe Theory* — This theory has been proposed by Orgel (1963). According to this theory, an accumulation of errors in the amino acid sequence in proteins, specially errors that affect the specifically of enzymes needed for protein synthesis, will result in further mistakes could occur during transcription of mRNA. Recently provided certain evidences in favour of this theory. They could shorten the life-span of adult fruit-flies by feeding a variety of amino acid analogues substitute phenylalanine and methonine respectively in the protein and interfere with the functions of proteins. Holliday has also detected abnormal forms of enzymes in ageing fibroblasts, while others have observed reduced specific activities of some enzymes isolated from aged organisms. Certain scientists even have speculated that errors are not the result of blind chance but are purposefully programmed probably by the "ageing genes". Regarding Error Theory, the Encyclopaedia observes "Orgel developed a model for biological ageing that is dependent upon a decrease in the fidelity of protein synthesis. In this way an accumulation of errors is thought to occur in enzyme synthesis systems such that faulty proteins would be specified leading to decrements in cell function. Evidence both for and against this hypothesis has been obtained, although there is currently (1976) a greater preponderance of negative data".

(xi) *Neuro-Hormonal Theory* — It states that brain is the biological clock, which determines ageing. The ageing is due to changes in the parts of CNS (Central Nervous System) which regulate the functioning of endocrine glands. Flinch suggested that the abnormal secretion of neuro-hormones from brain causes hormonal imbalance and real functioning of body parts and induce ageing. So there is a brain-endocrine master plan controlling the ageing process.

(xii) *Redundant Message Theory* — This is partly based on error accumulation. Medyedev suggests an interesting alternative hypothesis. His conceptions based on the fact that within each cell the genetic message is written in very highly redundant fashion.

(xiii) *Programmed Genetic Events* —According to this notion the switching on or off of genes during development process also determine age changes, i.e., age changes like developmental changes are programmed into the orginal pool of genetic information and are "played out" in an orderly sequence just as developmental changes are. The greying of hair is not taken as some kind of disease but a natural developmental change of time. It is a highly pre-diseable event that occur later in life after the genetic expression of myriad and other programmed developmental events that occur in orderly sequence.

(xiv) *Meantime to Failure* — Just like machines which has a life of particular period or years, similar is the case of human beings. Failure of cell function may occur at predictable times that are dependent upon the fidelity of the synthesising machinery and the degree of perfection of cellular repair systems. Since biological systems do not appear to function perfectly and indefinitely, we are led to the conclusion that the ultimate death of a cell or loss of function is genetically programmed and has "a meantime of failure". The meantime to failure may be applicable to a single cell, tissue, organ, or the intact animal itself. It is proposed that the genetic apparatus simply runs out of accurate programmed information that might in different "meantimes to failure" for all the dependent biological systems. The existence of different life spans for all species may be the reflection of mere perfect repair systems in those animals of greater longevity.

Can there be some Anti-Ageing Measure

This leads to the question, can there be any way to increase life span or to delay ageing as well to the question, if there are any anti-ageing ways and methods and if so, what are they? The average span of life is taken as 100 years. With the development of medical science, average life span has increased but as yet it has reached not upto 100 years. Some people die prematurely due to some specific diseases, like cancer, heart attack, TB and many other unexpected reasons, like accident, cholera, etc. In advanced years, several diseases crop up by way of biological disorders. But even if the medical science becomes capable to cure some such diseases like cancer, TB, cardiac arrest, etc., the life span may increase from the present life expectancy to 0.1 to 0.5 years not more, and of course, not 100 years. Thus biomedical research may help man in two ways (1) reduce or eliminate the particular cause of death, e.g., TB, cancer, heart attacks, cholera, encephalitis, etc., and (2) to address itself specifically to underlying non-disease related fundamental biological changes that occur with time. These are really speaking not diseases but are basic biological changes that result in those physiological decrements characteristic of ageing and upon which are often superimposed an increasing vulnerability to disease. Such an approach does not directly concern itself with efforts to increase human life expectation but rather to extend what appears to be a fixed human life-span.

Some of the gerontologists say that from a particular age, administration of less calorie food may be given/allowed to the individual person/animal which may be called under-nutrition level food, but not to the level of mal-nutrition level food. Experiments on animals in this concept has proved successful and such gerontologists have claimed that longevity can be enhanced by 50 per cent, as also that would lead to the "stretching out of the developmental stage, infancy, puberty, maturity, adulthood and ageing simply occur at later than usual point of time, so that the total life span is increased". Thus the under-nutritional diet may be very useful.

But attached to the above is the question of the quality of life one wants to live. Man wants to enjoy life, not only to linger it to some extent. If less calories diet are usually taken, enjoyment of life would be hampered, so nobody would like to stick to this formula of quantitative life or longevity at the cost of qualitative life. This type would be hardly accepted to all.

Some psychologists say that life span can be increased by regulation of hours of sleep but even of what the psychologist have said be granted, then it would hardly extend the total life span upto 100 years. Some psychologists say that more hours of sleep would be useful for longevity, but in the *Gita*, it has been said that when the common man sleeps in the night, the *yogi* remain wakeful and *yogis* live a longer life. Now which of the two should be adopted, it is difficult to say.

Some men say that life span can be enhanced by less sexual contact in life, sexual contacts may be limited for the purpose of having a child or two, not more, this would increase life. The Indian theory says that less sex contact is an important factor to increase life and reduce ageing process. (Loss of more semen leads to lessening of life itself.)

Tampering of Biological Clock

Some biological and gerontological researches have devised a theory which is called "*Tampering of biological clock*". There is a sharp difference between disease-oriented biomedical research and gerontological research. The question with the gerontologists is not to make a person free from a disease, but the question before them is, whether the "resolution" of the physiological decrements of old age will benefit the individual or society as whole. If it be granted that the biologists would become capable of eliminating old age related physiological decrements and no control were established over the biological clock itself, the result might be a society "whose members would live full physically vigorous, youthful lives until their 100th birthday at which time they would die" but this would further have the consequence that with the tampering of biological clock, or learning to tamper the biological clocks, it would lead to lingering of the sufferings of the period of infirmity of old age. One might enjoy particular age, say young age for some more time period, but this enjoyment of youth would lead to further enhancement of old by the number of years the youth had been extended. For example, one has extended youth starting from 20 years by 10-20 years, it would lead to increase in 10 years to 20 years of old and infirmity age, thus the span of old age with infirmity and suffering would then be 30 years. In this condition who will like to live 30 years of infirmity life than to increase youth. Further, it is difficult to ascertain what age would be most productive age which has to be extended. In fact, man is productive throughout life, so no specific period may be fixed prior hand as most productive age. So tempering of biological clock would really be tragic for the individual as well as the society, it would be tragic and detrimental to individual since it would increase his physical sufferings of his infirmity periods and it would further be tragic for the society since the young members of the family of such man would have to bear a lot of suffering in carrying on the liability of the infirm person and suffer hellish life of endless burdens, penury due to cost of medicine and health care.

In view of these, it is not possible to prescribe a foolproof theory of restricting, arresting and stopping age and the biological/ physiological/ gerontological scientists/researches have still to find out some foolproof measure for retarding, restricting, delaying or stopping old age. Old age is permanent phenomena of life, by no measure an evading problem. If youth comes man feels that childhood has gone far behind but when youth comes old age is not far behind. Old age has not only to be faced, but to be lived and lived in sportsman spirit with no other remedy in sight. Can we seek the remedy in our *Yoga* science and Ayurveda? This requires an elaborate discussion and certainly a somewhat fruitful one.

Chapter 11

Ageing : A Conceptual Analysis

Shiva Nath Prasad

It is very difficult to give a precise and exact definition of ageing, though we can describe about an old person, merely by looking at an old man from a distance. We can see a man and can easily say, that he is an old man. By what criteria, we declare that this is an old man, *prima facie*, by physical appearance only, I or anyone, can declare that such and such man appears to be an old man. In the very sight of an old man, we find some outward factors by which standard or criteria we can say that a certain man appears to be an old man. We only see a man and since his age is not written on his forehead, so we cannot say what is his age or how old he is. Age cannot be adequate criteria for old person. We only see the physical appearance and that itself gives a clue to declare that he is an old. There are certain signs which differentiated anyone as an old man, as distinguished from a young man or child. An old man's vision is reduced, he cannot see right, he develops cataract in the eyes, which gives less or disturbed vision. His teeth decays, breath falls down and he cannot chew food rightly in the manner a young man chew. His cheek sinks in. The walls between and around the eyeball, also sink down. His hairs get greyed. His memory is lost. His energies also get dwindled. These are the physical signs of an old man. It is difficult to say at what age one starts becoming old, though age is also a physical factor. In the holy book *Ramcharita Manas* of Tulsidas, what is ordinarily called an old age has been termed *chauthapam*, the word *Chauthapan*, means fourth stage. According to the *āshram vyavasthā* in India, *chauthāpan* is the stage of fourth *āshram,* i.e., *sanyās āshram*. The *King Dasrath* was very much in grief, when he did not have any son even in the stage of *chauthapan*. The *Ramcharita Manas* says that when Dasrath saw his face in the mirror and found that the hairs of the head behind his ears have greyed, he felt that he has gone old and so he was filled with anxiety for getting a son for transferring his crown. Thus in the Rāmāyan, one criteria of old age has been greying of hairs behind the ears. There is one more criteria of old age for the kings. It has been said that when the crown fitted on the head starts loosening, i.e. when the crown does not fit tightly on the head, the signs of oldness becomes clear. This means that in the old age, due to the shrinkage of the skin and flesh of the head, the crown fails to fit tightly on the head and this in itself shows that he has developed signs of decay and the decayed state is a symbol of old age. Thus we can see by the eyes and can tell that this is an old man but age cannot be taken as sufficient determinant of old age, nor have we any sort of measuring rod for age. Moreover, there are persons who look tired, deteriorated, depressed at a very early age in the very youth, while there are some, who though grown in years, do not show signs of old age, due to his energeticness, his boldness of approach, etc. There are some people, whose hairs start greying at a very early age, even in the childhood stage, while there are some whose hairs do not grey even at a fairly old age. There are several physical factors, depending upon the individual, which show less signs of ageing than others. There are several psychological factors which also work. A depressed and frustrated man seems to look older in their youth, though other, who is psychologically satisfied from the life, he is spending energetic life look young even at a fairly ripe age. Thus we cannot say definitely, at what age one becomes older or at what age, he starts getting old. Further, the process of transition from one stage, i.e., childhood to youth or from youth to old age is a natural change and a very slow process and it is difficult to measure the differences from one stage to another stage. Though from the very childhood, one grows day-by-day, but we cannot see the growth from the physical vision. It is all an inward, natural and imperceptible growth process and no one can know the growth day-by-day, not only the others who see, but even the person himself in question cannot mark the difference. Of course, one can mark the difference after 10 years or so, when there is a large scale of wear and tear of the cells of the body. In the measurement of, or determination of old age, two most important factors are involved, which are quantitative factors and qualitative factors, which may roughly correspond to the quality of life one passes, the years one has passed over. While the quantitative factor refers to lapse of years in one's life, which is a physical measuring rod, the qualitative factors involve the psychological factors, the environment in which he lives, the familial background in which the person lives, the financial status, in which the person lives: these factors affect the mental make-up of the man, too much, the ageing problems depend upon these psychological factors. It is said that the "face is the index of mind", but the physical state also clearly reflects on the face. There is no water tight compartmentalisation between the physical and psychological realm. Both the psychological and physical realm go side-by-side, so it is said in a well known proverb "a sound mind in a sound body", i.e., if the physical frame of a man is frail, the mental factors are not less protected, rather the physical and psychological factors go equally together, the one effecting the other, the one interacting and reacting creeping into the other. Human beings have not as yet devised a common mechanical measuring tool to weigh or measure either the process of ageing or the transformation of young into old age or old age itself. In this state of affairs, we have to find out or to search out a conceptual intellectual schemata or framework to resolve the impasse and look out for a philosophical study of ageing, which nonetheless, is not a present problem but a problem for all times. Since the very old days, even since the very inception of human race, men used to take birth, to become young, to become old and one day breath his last. The stages of life, called better, childhood, youth, old age and death are ever-recurrent problems and despite all advancement in the medical sciences, up till now, no one has been able to find out a medicine or drug which could stop this process once for all. Further, it is also very difficult to say, that soon our medical science would be able to research one potent drug or medicine, which would arrest old age and keep a child always a child and young man ever young, or old aged returning to childhood or youth. It would be a red letter day for the medical science to invent such a medicine. Only there are some mystics or mystic poets like Henry Vaughn who has said I may return from old age to childhood.

It has been said that old age, disease, death, etc., are perennial problems, which had engaged the mind of man, ever since the inception of life. It is known to all that Buddha, saw an old man, a diseased man and a dead body and these sights filled his heart with grief. Like the medical scientists of the day, he also was filled with the idea of researching or finding out the ways to stop disease, stop old age and avoid death. Buddha was an affluent man, he was a king and had all resources to avail of a kingly life. His father left for him enough of wealth and material possession which could go well for his whole life. But Buddha was a ponderous man, his mind was filled with unrest at the sight of a perfectly diseased man, an old man and a dead body. He was all through worried how to avoid all these or rescue such man. He wanted to find out a panacea of such ills of life. He had a beautiful wife, a beautiful child, he could have enjoyed the pompous mundane pleasures, but one night, he was so much overwhelmed that he left his wife, child and the home and set out to discover the remedy of these mundane sufferings, so that these could be stopped once for all. His heart was full of milk of human kindness. He spent his long periods living the life of recluse or *sannyasi*, doing *tapa*, performing penance, torturing his body. His long *tapas* resulted in sudden enlightenment under the Bodhi tree and he came out with panacea of the ills of life, which lay not in torturing the body, but by overcoming all desires or *trisna* or *tanhā* as it is called in Pali. He found out the panacea of all ills of life, *nirvana* or salvation. He gave the four Arya *satyas*, that there is misery in life, there is a cause of misery, there is a cessation of misery, and there is a way to the cessation of misery. He gave his theory of dependent origination or *pratitya samutpāda*, then the *dvādash nidāna.* He gave his theory of *prajna*, *shila*, *samadhi*, *karunā, maitri*, etc. Buddha really worked like a great scientist in the laboratory of his life and found out the remedy of the ills of life not by combining certain medicinal herbs or chemicals either in pill form or aqueous form, but in the form of controlling the meanderings of mind in moving from one object to another, in trying to fulfil this desire or that, rather by perfectly getting rid all desires, which are the root cause of birth and death, the endless cycle of birth and death, which are themselves pure misery, birth is misery, death is misery, even this whole life is misery. So he said first strike out the desire and you will be set free from the trammels of misery. The *Dhammapada* says, first kill the enemy of desire.

Not only did the Buddha strive towards the goal of removing the miseries of life, but all the systems of Indian philosophy have tried to find out the common goal of getting relieved of the burden of misery, each in their own way. The *yoga* system strives to attain this by checking the meandering of minds, *chitta vṛtti nirodha*, the *Samkhya* by attaining discriminatory knowledge of the two different, but opposed principles of *purusa* and *prakṛti*. The nyaya system seeks the same in some other way, using different remarks.

There is an anecdote with regard to the great writer and thinker Emerson. Emerson was celebrating his sixtieth birthday, he was asked by one man, what is your age? And he said "Three hundred sixty years". The man could not believe it, he felt as if Emerson could not perhaps hear his question. So he repeated this question twice, thrice and more, and Emerson gave the same reply time and again. The person asked once again, I could not hear, "Emerson said, You have fully heard what I have said, i.e., three hundred sixty years." The man said, "I cannot believe it. You must be joking.... You don't look more than sixty years old, but said Emerson, "my consciousness is six times more than sixty. I count my age according to my intelligence, not according to my body, because I am not the body, I am my intelligence". This reply is an example of the growing old but intelligence growing far ahead the age of the body. This speaks of growing down of the body but growing up of the intelligence, consciousness, awareness and wisdom. If wisdom be, age is left far behind, a statement similar to the statement of the great English poet "If spring comes winter is left far behind". There is a great difference between growing in age, growing old and the intelligence going upwards, i.e. growing up. Rajneesh tried to understand this fact of 'ageing' with the help of two words "growing old and growing up."

A great poet has said, "we live in deeds, not in years, since the daffodil (a flower) has a small span of life of one day, it falls in the night, it is born in the morn, still it is a "flower of light", while an oak tree lives for hundred years, but all its life is hackneyed it gives no benefit to anyone. Similar is the poetry of Rahim, the Hindi poet, who has said, बड़ा हुआ तो क्या हुआ जैसे ताड़ खजूर, पंथी को छाया नहीं फल लागे अति दूर, The palm and khajur tree grow up in height, they go too high, but they don't either give relief, by giving shadow for the travellers from heat of the sun nor do they give their fruit to man, since the fruits grow in such height that it is impossible to pluck the fruits from such heights nor are the fruits so tasteful. This is growing up, but for nothing except a dull life, profitless, useless even for a common man. It is really going down, not growing up. And Rajneesh says, "Growing old is not of any worth, even animal does it, it needs no intelligence. Growing up is different experience. Growing old is horizontal, growing up is vertical, it is leading to heights, it leads you to depths". Unnatural as it may appear, there are person of seventy years of age, but their mind seems to be of the like of a child of seven years. The mind of such a man is kept retarded, otherwise just as the body of a man grows, the physiology of man grows, the mental age ought to follow simultaneously, but the mind plays the havoc. The retarded mind does not let the man grow up with the growth of the body. Here the age of the body is growing up, while the mind is growing down, it is moving inversely, backwards not in any forward direction. This growing down, being retarded mentally makes man dull, desireless, it cuts life from the sap of life and man remains merely a frail structure full of ageing, mistrust, distrust, disharmony, full of anguish, negativity, passivity, sluggishness, lethargy, fickleness, disgust, quarrelsomeness. This is the picture in general of 'old age' or ageing. But to Rajneesh, this is not the true picture of an old man or a grown up man, whose mind should have grown up with age. This is one-sided picture of old age and a destructive way of looking at things in all its negativity. This negative attitude has to go outright, so that a rosy picture of old age can be presented, thus taking old age not as a curse, but as a wisdom-giving age, serving as light unto others. Rajneesh will say that old age should be taken with positive attitude rather than wrapt rolled round in negativity, passivity, anguish, flimsiness, vacuity, making the end of life a curse, a sin, a misfortunes a downfall, misfortune, destiny turned inimical and adverse. This is a narrow-necked picture of one of the most important periods of life, the old age. Old age must show signs of wisdom.

Really speaking, according to Rajneesh, life is a regale, a celebration and this celebration should not only begin with the birth of a child, it must continue till death and even after death, because death is not something of an enemy of man, it is a great rejuvinator, it gives fresh life, like changing of old cloth with a new one, when the old cloth gets torn or worn out, as in the *Gita*, death offers opportunity for a new life. So death should not be taken as sickness, as fearful, rather a comforter as the poet Rabindranath Tagore, who has compared death with the Supreme Lord Shyam or Kṛṣṇa. Vinovaji took death as a great and unfailing friend *Param Sakhā*. Rajneesh accepts the views of the *Gita*, the changing of old cloth, in the form of a worn out body, at the time of death for getting a new cloth of body, a new body for further engagement and celebration, life for him is a celebration, not a gloom or despair, it is a game, funfair, fun feast, not a wailing, sobbing, repenting, revenging, restraining, but regaling attitude to death will also be no less rejoicing and merriful and mystifying. Let death be also a celebration and playful as all life is.

Life is a gift, a bounty. Man is born to achieve it. He may miss it, it depends on him to miss it or to make it. He may go on breathing, go on eating, he can go on growing old, he can go on moving towards the grave — but this is not life. This amounts to gradual death, from cradle to the grave, dying at an average age of seventy or so. Millions of people are dying everyday, everybody sees it. This slow pace of death becomes an imitation for everyone in thought at least, and the real mission of life is missed. Life is *virāt* says the Hindu *Sastras*. There is a great mission in this life, man is *amṛtasya putrah*, he has to achieve divinity in this very life, the Vedantic teachings are harping upon this fact, the *Upanisads* are repeatedly saying this. Swami Vivekanand and Sri Aurobindo have harped upon this Vedantic approach: A baby is born, he grows, he becomes a child, he grows, becomes young and he grows, he becomes old. Every day after the birth of a child is a day nearer to his death. A child becomes of five years. This means that his death is nearer five years. He has spent five years approaching towards death. This approach of life as hastening to death, would make life unliveable, inactive, pessimistic. Life should be taken to be growing like the tree, going upwards in height, but not only upwards but also going deeper in its roots, to such depths which can balance the height of the entire weight of the branches, trunk of tree, otherwise the whole tree would break down, fall down.

So the mission of life is to realise only own being, one's own existence and if this prime mission is not realised, life becomes a worse, stale, stinking worth not a farthing. The Indian *sastras* speak of identifying the *atman* with Brahman and for the fulfilment of this great mission, life should be endless toil, earning bread by sweet of one's brow, eating one's honest farthing and also toiling to achieve the highest goal of salvation, freedom and eternity, *moksa*, though Buddha did not use the word '*moksa*', but he gave his new word '*nirvana*' meaning 'blowing out of the light', Life to him is an incessant flowing stream; birth, youth, old age, and consequent death are only stages of life, the cuts and intervals of life for simple moments. All life, all existence is continuous. Death is not the end. Death is also a bead in the garland of life, a chain which moves round in small stead, in stages, in circularity, no bead of garland can be separated, it moves on and on, there is nothing like the last bead or the first. Buddha's philosophy of Dependent Origination, his *Pratitya Samutpada* theory, emphasises on this fact. Buddha says to achieve *nirvana* by one's own labour. "Work out thy salvation". This means that life has deeper missions, old age or death does not deter this achieving the supreme end of life. This sort of thing, is an approach which can be said to be "growing up" approach in terms of Rajneesh. Old age which turns into death is only a stage prior to death, and death is the greatest illusion there is, according to Nietzsche and Rajneesh, and they will say "for growing up, just watch a tree. As the tree goes up, its roots are growing down, deeper. There is a balance, the higher the tree goes the deeper the roots will go. You cannot have a tree 150 feet high with small roots; they could not support such a huge tree". In life, growing up means growing deep within yourself—that's where your roots are". This growing up and growing deep down, both taken and combined in simultaneity really fulfils the mission of life, the mission of existence. The two words of Rajneesh "growing up and growing down" are important words to explain the whole life and existence. Sri Aurobindo also says that the whole world is cyclic process, and death is but a stage, not the final halt, similarly old age is also a stage, it should not be taken to be negative of life itself, but a stage of development, not the end. To Rajneesh, old age or death is not retrogression, a backward drive but a progression, a forward, ongoing drive. Old age should signify growing up in wisdom rather growing down in the form of gripping in misery.

The animals are also gifted with life, but they only grow old. Only animals can grow old, animals are capable if growing old. But "growing up" is the peculiar and singular prerogative of man or human beings, of which animals are not at all capable of. Animals are not capable of mind, or intelligence, so growing old does not remove or increase anything in animals. But the human beings have intelligence and he is capable of wisdom, so with growing in age, he accomplishes wisdom and that wisdom or *jnana* will lead him to cross the ocean of existence to eternity, endless freedom, to absolute blissful stage of *sat*, *chit* and *anand*. Our ancient sages have roared undauntedly "know thyself", i.e., knowledge or wisdom leads to immortality, they also say that only that knowledge or wisdom is to be taken as wisdom, which is capable of leading one to immortality सा विद्या वा विमुक्तये", that is *vidya* which brings immortality. In this context Rajneesh says, "growing up means moving every moment deeper into the principle of life; it means going farther away from death not towards death. The deeper you go into life, the more you understand the immortality within you. You are moving away from death, a moment comes when you can see that death is nothing but changing clothes, or changing houses, changing forms — nothing dies, nothing can die".

We live from moment to moment and die. In sleep we die to the world, in waking we awake to the world. The *Purusa sukta* illustrates the metaphysical validity of the ethics of 'die to live' it illustrates the fundamental paradox that all life is like Nature, a "resurrection", a coming into life out of death; for, death is not the last phase, but a condition of the enduring renewal of life; the willing sacrifice is a proof of his Law. When in youth, he sacrifices himself for the offspring, it is an obligation, but when he becomes old, it is the obligation of the offspring to sacrifice his pleasure for the pleasure of the elder parents or elder kith and kin. It is a reciprocal give and take, a religious and obligatory duty. The old person may be taken in this light in accordance with Indian spiritual and religious culture, not in accordance with Western Culture which speaks or pleads for nuclear family, adopt individualistic and pragmatic stance.

In dying to our daily pleasure of now, is also living pleasure of the elderly people, a give-and-take process rather than wasting exercise. For making old age mirthful and merrisome, it is most essential that the man has lived his childhood and youth in perfect enjoyful mode, living from moment to moment enjoy each bit of life, each moment leaving no scope for remorse, repentance and a feeling of having not availed of the joys, he ought to have enjoyed. The repression of past joys, even sex-enjoyment or even other desires would leave a trail of unsatisfaction, this repressed satisfaction brings the old age an age of frustration, misery helplessness, whimsicalness, etc., and all these would make man old even before he attains old. So if a man lives from moment to moment, his old age would not reflect old age, old age would become happy old and will lead to happy death, unfearful death, unafraid death.

According to Rajneesh, man is an individual, and this "individuality" is indivisible. It has no layers, upward layer to downward like the layers of onion. The individual is one whole, it is unbreakable, it is one whole, it is a unity, a harmony. A real grown up person is one indivisible, not like onion which has layers and go on removing the layers, the end would be nothing. Take a sheet of mica, there are layers upon layers, and when layers after layers are removed in the end nothing remains. Personality, according to Rajneesh, has layers, it is imitative, individuality is innovative. A person may be loving father, a jealous husband, a hypocritic friend. All these are layers of his personality but individuality is death of personality. Buddha said, take a drop from the sea, from bottom, from upward, from such north, east, west, the taste would be same, salty. Similarly a really grown up person is one, he is always the same, formal he is the same, informal, he is the same, in love, in logic, in society, in privacy, he is the same one and this sameness says Rajneesh is his, growing-up-ness. His centre has become his periphery, so in and out, there is no distinction, he is oneness. An un-grown person behaves variously in different situations, his superficial layer acts actively and his behaviour becomes hypocritical while a really grown up man is true to all, in all circumstances, he is steadfast, unwavering something akin to *dhirbuddhi* or *sthiti prajna* of the *Gita*. He has nothing to hide or expose, he is one and uniform, he is unique, so individual. An ungrown person behaves like a child. Though he is of 60 years or behaves like a fool or like an insane man.

Growing old does not mean that the man has attained maturity. To become old and still remain childish is much embarrassing. Meditation, says Rajneesh, is needed in order to bring a total transformation in man. Merely accumulating experience is not much. Accumulation of experience may make a man well informed about many things, but information is information, it cannot bring transformation. Only meditation can bring transformation, growing in age do not bring maturity. It can make man ripe in knowledge, grown in wisdom.

"The body is a momentary phenomena, it is like foam, it exists for the time being, it looks so beautiful. And if the sun has risen, around the foam can be created a rainbow.... looks like diamonds, looks so white and so pure. But if you take it in your hands, it starts disappearing. Only your hands are left wet, that's all. So is the case of the body. It looks beautiful, but death is growing in it, death is hiding it, old age is hiding in it, old age is waiting there. It is only a question of time."

According to Rajneesh, it is strange phenomena in man that what is superficial layer in him comes first, the real nature remains hidden and submerged. You scratch a person a little and all his grown-up-ness would be gone, and he will behave like a child or a fool of first order. The great difficulty with old man is that he grows old, but his childishness still remains. This is most embarrassing. For a child to be childish is not an embarrassing, but a child behaving like old man, or an old man behaving like a child is disturbing.

There is a general apathy and disgust about an old man, nobody likes his company, not even his child. The reason for such situation is not old age, but the magic of his desires have faded, he behaves like rock, like stony attitude of indifference. He becomes callous. He cannot tolerate anyone loving, he is away with his condemning eyes, revengeful eyes, what he failed in his own life comes for him as condemnable from others. If an old had not get fully enjoyed life, he wants that other should also not enjoy, he feels jealous of others often revengeful. He feels that he is dying and the other people are loving how could it be. The other people enjoying becomes unacceptable for the old man. The unlived of youth penetrates into old age, old age becomes dirty, ugly. Sex becomes cerebral, not genital. In youth love ends in bed, such affair is impossible for old person. Youth is feverish, old is understanding old age has already passed through feverish warmth of young age, so Rajneesh says that old age is not ageing, but wisdom too and you have to pass through the fire of youth to become pure gold old age.

Old person often cunning, insincere, dishonest and this body to apathy. Rajneesh remarks, every child is a 'warrior and every old man is a businessman', and he elaborates, abusiveness means calculating cunning mind, child's mind is simple, not cunning, it is difficult to find an old man who is not cunning. A warrior jumps into war, there is no time for him to think. Old man has time in plenty for thought, he has experience.

Rajneesh distinguishes between two concepts "freedom from" and "freedom for". "Freedom from" is a reaction, it is ego asserting as freedom from slavery. Freedom is reactionary, not an understanding. In 1917, the Russians revolted against the Czar, their idea of freedom was negative. 'Freedom for' is positive and far better of love for music, it is not against, but for. The first type of people becomes politician, the second type becomes a poet, artist, painter, dancer, musician. There is a third kind of freedom without 'for' or 'from', it is transcendental freedom, it is real freedom, love, *nirvan*, that freedom is truth. It is blessedness, it is a stage after the ego has died, unless your mind turns inward, becomes "meditation", you cannot be grown-up.

The real reason behind distrust of youth to older people is the clash of ego of the two. If the ego is gone, then there is no problem. So Rajneesh emphasizes too much for erasing the ego.

Chapter 12

Animal Rights : Ethical Perspective

Devarakonda Balaganapathi

We are the living graves of murdered beasts,
Slaughtered to satisfy our appetites.
We never pause to wonder at our feasts,
If animals, like man, can possibly have rights.
We pray on Sundays that we may have light
To guide our footsteps on the path we tread.
We're sick of war; we do not want to fight;
The thought of it now fills our hearts with dread,
And ye....we gorge ourselves upon the dead.
Like carrion crows, we live and feed on meat,
Regardless of the suffering and pain
We cause by doing so. If thus we treat
Defenseless animals for sport or gain,
How can we hope in this world to attain
The peace we say we are so anxious for.
We pray for it, o'er hetacombs of slain,
To God, while outraging the moral law.
Thus cruelty begets its offspring ...WAR !

George Bernard Shaw

The present day world could be viewed as; (i) Natural world, where natural law prevails and where humans are one of the many species of animals that live; and (ii) Artificial world or social world that is created by man for himself, where man-made laws prevail. In the natural world both humans and animals have equal rights. The situation is rather complex in the artificial world, where everything happens to help, support and sustain man in accomplishing his goals. Man, in this world, is supreme. This made him now, though he was once a part of nature, alien to nature. He, further, started using the non-human beings and things for his own selfish purposes. Animals are one of the non-human beings that became means for human accomplishments. Today, we see different kinds of animals being used at different places for different reasons, all to accomplish the goals of man. The 'exploitation of the animals', as Peter Singer (1993) call it, is of different kinds. Animals are used for food; for testing the medicine in the laboratories; for giving enjoyment in circus and movies, and also for commercial purposes like selling animals for petting to selling the skin and other parts of the animals as decoratory items. In India superstitious beliefs also contribute for the animal killing. Sacrificing animals in the name of gods is still persistent in many places. Even the basic right of the animals like right to life is also not recognized in the human society.

In this kind of a situation it is necessary to analyze the rights of humans themselves. Of course, man has social, cultural and political rights, which protect him from other human beings. However, does he have any right over the other beings of the world? As man has a fundamental right to live — in the same way, is it not fair to think that animals, which are his co-beings also have a right to live? This chapter, in trying to explicate the problems involved in articulating the rights of the non-human beings, questions the very right of man over the non-human world. The aim of this chapter is to elevate the status of animals rather than to lower the status of the humans. My argument is for limiting the rights of man and extending his duties to nature in general and animals in particular.

I

Let us look at the Western philosophical traditions to locate the place of animals in the human world. In the West it was traditionally believed that animals were made for the human use. This idea, familiar from the Old Testament elaborated by a long line of Christian thinkers and it also formed part of Aristotle's world view. Aristotle in his discussion on 'On Soul' in *Nichomachean Ethics* thought that 'nature does everything for a purpose', and so, just as plants exist to provide food for animals, animals exist to provide food and other 'aids in life' for humans. He believed that animals lack reason and belief. Aquinas emphasized that 'it was God himself who provided the animals for human use'. Therefore, he said, 'it is not wrong for man to make use of them, by killing or in any other way whatever'. One might think that we have a duty to be kind to them out of simple charity. But Aquinas insisted that this is not so. He said, 'charity does not extend to irrational creatures'. Thus, giving less significance to non-human animals and privileged status to the humans by the tradition, rests on two important arguments. First one is given by Aristotle, that is, 'humans alone are rational'; another one is based on the religious faith that man alone was made in the image of God.

This bias towards humans in the Western philosophical tradition was followed even in the modern period. Whereas traditional thought deprived animals from reason and privileged birth from God, modern thought deprived animals from thought and language. Descartes, who is considered to be the father of modern philosophy, states that language use is creative and is unbound in scope. Hence, though "magpies and parrots are able to utter words just like ourselves' this is mechanical, 'a movement of mere nature' rather than a sign of thought. He considered nonhumans animals as biological robots and simply physical creatures which are incapable of sensation and pain. Thus, Descartes argues that animals do not have thought 'for the word is the sole sign and the only certain mark of the presence of thought hidden and wrapped up in the body'. Since animals do not have thoughts they do not have 'real feeling', for 'real feeling' involves propositional content and animals are incapable of propositional content because they do not have language.

Immanual Kant, most influential German philosopher of the modern time, in his *Ground Work for a Metaphisics of Morals* puts *persons* at the centre of morality and argues that treating *persons* merely as a means to our own ends is wrong. He argued that since animals are not 'persons', morality cannot be attributed to them. To be a person, for him, is to be an autonomous being, and should have the capacity to act for reasons and also to be able to reason about its reasons. Since nonhuman animals do not have these capacities, they are beyond the pale of morality. However, it is interesting to note that Kant did recommend that animals should be treated nicely not out of moral obligation, but to avoid developing insensitive character in us.

According to Social contract theory, which was developed in the seventeenth century, morality is the product of an agreement among the members of society. Each of us agrees to follow certain rules on the condition that others do the same. We have no such obligations to those who are not part of the agreement. Nonhuman animals, which are incapable of entering into contracts, are not part of the agreement. Therefore, we have no moral obligations to them.

Wittgenstein, one of the most prominent philosophers of the twentieth century, in his *Philosophical Investigations (1953)* though appears to think that animals have sensations, emotions, intentions and first order beliefs, however, denies that animals have power to stimulate pain, to talk to themselves, or have attitudes about future events. Behaviourists, like Quine, regard ascribing thoughts to animals as an 'essential dramatic idiom'. We imagine ourselves in the animal's place and say what thoughts we would have were we the animal. According the Davidson, if an animal has a thought, then this thought must occur in a network of beliefs. This follows from Davidson's holism which he takes from Quine; thoughts or beliefs come in webs, they cannot occur simply. In order to have a network of beliefs an animal must have a concept of belief. This is because having a network of beliefs requires the ability to distinguish between someone holding a sentence to be true and the sentence actually being true. But having the concept of belief requires having language — for Davidson believes that this concept only arises in the context of linguistic interpretation. Since no animals have language they do not have the concept of belief. Since they do not have the concept of belief they do not have networking of beliefs. Hence they do not have beliefs at all.

In this way, all these modern arguments presuppose a close connection between thought and language. They suppose that language is a necessary condition for having thoughts. To conclude, by following the western philosophical tradition we have no obligations towards animals. Nevertheless, we may have moral obligations *concerning* them, but those obligations are to other people. We ought not, for example, poison somebody else's pet, for the same reason that we ought not destroy somebody else's property.

However, there are few exceptions in the modern philosophy in support of the animal rights. Jeremy Bentham (1749), Utilitarian philosopher of modern times, showed the first sign of concern towards animals when he said, I quote:

> The day may come when the rest of the animal creation may acquire those rights which never could have been withholden from them but by the hand of tyranny. The French have already discovered that the blackness of the skin is no reason why a human being should be abandoned without redress to the caprice of a tormentor. It may one day come to be recognized that the number of legs, the villosity of the skin, or the termination of the *os sacrum* are reasons equally insufficient for abandoning a sensitive being to the same fate. What else is it that should trace the insuperable line? Is it the faculty of reason, or perhaps the faculty of discourse? But a full-grown horse or

> dog is beyond comparison, a more rational, as well as a more conversable animal, than an infant of a day or a weak or even a month, old. But suppose they were otherwise, what would it avail? The question is not, Can they *reason*? nor Can they *talk*? but Can they *suffer*? (1749:311)

Bentham, thus brought *suffering to the centre of morality to conclude nonhuman animals into the moral sphere.* Continuing this trend, few scholars argued that there is continuity across the species. Darwin, for instance, demonstrated that humans are not set apart from other animals, but are related to them by evolutionary descent. Our bones and muscles are but modified versions of the ape's bones and muscles — they are similar because we inherited them from the same ancestors. The same is true of our rational faculties. Man is not the only rational animal, for other animals also possess a degree of rationality. Since our brains developed from a common source, Darwin went so far as to declare that there is no fundamental difference between man and the higher mammals in their mental faculties (1859:35). He regarded cruelty to animals, along with slavery as one of the two great moral failings.

Landmark in the history of animal rights came in the year 1975, when Australian philosopher Peter Singer published his book *Animal Liberation,* with the basic moral message that 'All animals are equal'. He argued that though our shared morality protects human animals from innumerable kinds of treatment we find intolerable, it is far less protective of nonhuman animals, and hence it is only partial. Singer brings nonhuman animals also under the moral framework by following the utilitarian principle that since we morally ought to maximize happiness and minimize suffering and as animals also can suffer, our calculations ought to include them as well. Since nonhuman animals, like human animals, also can experience both pleasure and pain, if it is wrong to cause human suffering to achieve a good that does not outweigh that suffering then it is wrong to cause nonhuman suffering to achieve such a good. However, the principle of utility has some limitations. If somebody, for instance, argues that the elimination of factory farms in which meat is produced would create havoc in the country's economy that utility is maximized by keeping them, then there can be no argument from the utilitarian point of view.

To avoid the limitations of the utilitarian argument, Tom Regan (1992) offers an alternative argument that, the focus of the moral concern is to avoid treating individual animals in certain ways regardless of the consequences. He argues that since all animals that are the experiencing subjects of their own lives have inherent value they should not be treated as mere things. For him, what makes eating meat or experimenting on animals wrong is not that the human benefit does not outweigh the animal suffering, but that such practices deny the inherent value of the animals involved.

Let us see what Indian tradition states about the animal rights. In contrast with the Western philosophical tradition of both classical and modern times, Indian philosophical tradition supports the animal rights from the beginning, at least indirectly, by enunciating the significance of the principle of *ahimsa* or non-injury. The *Vedas* which are earliest philosophical literature; *Dharmasastras* which contain the highest moral codes of conduct, and all the philosophical schools, both orthodox and heterodox, propagate *ahimsa* as the supreme principle of the ethical world. For instance, *Upanishads* considered love of brute creation, i.e., animals to be a great virtue. Kindness and compassion for all that has life on earth is a general feature of Indian ethics. *Yoga* school of philosophy, while explaining *niyama* which is one of the eight limbs of *yoga*, explicates *ahimsa* as one of the *niyamas* that an individual should follow in order to make himself prepared for the yogic *sadhana*. *Mahabharata* proclaims that non-injury is the highest virtue, when it says; *Ahimsa paramo dharmah.* Jainism and Buddhism, two prominent heterodox schools of Indian thought, base their whole ethical doctrines on the principle of *ahimsa*. The most fervent exponents of *ahimsa* as non-injury even to animals are Jainism. Vardhamana Mahavira, the twenty third *tirthankara*, insisted that we should not injure life whether in sport or in sacrifice. He says:

All beings hate pains
Therefore one should not kill them
This is the quintessence of wisdom, not
To kill anything.

This doctrine lead Jainas to most extraordinary practices like, sweeping of paths as one walks along and the wearing of gauze over one's mouth to avoid the accidental killing of any creature. They believed that all beings possess soul and spirit. They define *ahimsa* not as mere negative abstention, but as positive kindness to all creation. Buddhist concept of Mahakaruna propagates that all beings must be treated with equal respect. Buddha taught:

A brother ought not intentionally
To destroy the life of any being.
Not for our life would we ever intentionally
Kill a living being.

Thus, both the orthodox and heterodox schools of Indian philosophical thought given equal consideration to animals along with humans. *Bhagavadgita* (xiii. 27) says: *samam sarveshu bhuteshu tishtantham parameshwaram.* Which means, the God, who is the lord of all beings, stays in all the beings equally. This goes in contrast with the western philosophical tradition that only humans are born from the God and animals are not. According to the *Gita*, God is there in all the beings and there is no discrimination and special privilege to any being. Thus, equality of all beings is enunciated in the Indian tradition. Indian tradition teaches us to worship the nature. Even from the olden days we are worshippers of animals. Of course, it is true that, on the name of worship animals were used to be sacrificed in the *yagnas* and *yagas*. There was resistance from nastic traditions like Carvaka, Jainism and Buddhism to the animal sacrifices in the Vedic rituals. Slowly the animal sacrifice is substitute by breaking pumpkin and the like.

Belief in *karma sidhanta* and the 'doctrine of transmigration of soul' of Hinduism support animals, though from a homocentric perspective. The doctrine of *karma* states that the birth of a being depends on its past *karma*. Thus, the soul that is reincarnated as a non-human animal is a former human who is thereby punished for misdeeds. Though this is a homocentric doctrine, its implications for the treatment of non-human animals are more favourable than the Western homocentrism. As an extension to this, *ahimsa* has been interpreted to presuppose that a soul changes bodily identities through a succession of lives, unless and until ultimate enlightenment is obtained.

II

Since the present day world is homocentric and given rise to the speciesistic attitude, it is necessary to re-assess and understand the rights and duties in the larger context of man as a member of the natural world, which includes lot of nonhuman beings and nonliving things.

Let us start with discussing 'what rights are?'

Routledge Encyclopedia of Philosophy gives a widespread and well accepted view of rights as the 'ways of acting or of being treated that are beneficial to the right-holder.' That means the right-holder should have benefit in doing his actions and also being an object of others actions towards him. This implies, from the point of view of the right-holder, that (1) I have a right to act in a certain way; and (2) I have a right not to be treated in certain ways. Thus, rights presuppose a right-holder, who acts and who becomes an object of the treatment of others. This, further, presupposes a kind of equality between the right holders, since rights are applicable to all the members of the group without exception. If all the right-holders have equal rights, then how can the clash between the rights of different right-holders be solved? This problem necessitates the prevalence of certain limitations as well as corresponding duties to the rights. For instance, a right-holder's liberty presupposes another right-holder's limitations.

There are two ways of understanding rights; *natural* and

artificial. Natural rights are those that a being possesses by its birth. Artificial rights are those that are created by man, for the smooth running of his artificial human world. *Social rights, political rights and moral rights are the examples of artificial rights*, whereas basic right like *right to life is a natural right*, that every being on the earth could be said to possess.

How can we justify the rights? How did they come into existence?

(a) Few say, rights are practices that are established socially.
(b) Others say, they are claims—a right is a justified claim or principle of some sort.

(a) is social and political whereas (b) is moral involving the normative direction of the behaviour or corresponding obligations. *These two explanations are applicable only to artificial rights of the human beings.*

Traditionally, as indicated above, it is argued that only persons, who are self-conscious beings and who are aware of themselves as distinct entities with a past and future, can have rights. Since animals cannot be considered as persons, they cannot have rights. There were experiments in the modern period to see whether animals could be qualified as persons. Peter Singer argues that animals are also self-conscious beings and they have a sense of time. Pet animals such as dogs and cats have time sense and also division of time into days and weeks and years, if not in the same way as we do have. Animals possess the memory of the past and expectations about the future. They also form intentions and act on them. They have cooperative activity which requires planning. They have deceptive behaviour which shows that they are both self-conscious and have an awareness of the consciousness of another. Animals can have intentions and also act for a reason. These have been proved experimentally on apes.

Another argument that deprived animals from rights is that they do not have a language and, therefore, they cannot think.

Hence, beings which cannot reason or think cannot have rights. However, there are many species of animals that use language. Certainly many animals have some means of communication, whether it be melodious songs of the humpback whales or the howls and barks of the dogs. According to Singer, "there is nothing altogether inconceivable about a being possessing the capacity for conceptual thought without having a language and there are instances of animal behaviour that are extraordinarily difficult, if not downright impossible, to explain except under the assumption that the animals are thinking conceptually" (1993: 114). For instance, Singer (1993:111) mentions the efforts of American scientists Allen and Beatrice proved that Chimpanzees can learn the language. However, they cannot talk since they do not have vocal equipment needed to produce the sounds of human language. A chimpanzee by name Washoe learned to understand about 350 different signs and to use about 150 of them correctly. She could even put signs together to form simple sentences. It is interesting to note that Washoe adopted an infant Chimpanzee and began deliberately teaching him signs. Thus, it is argued that at least few higher animals can be qualified, if not all, as persons, having the sense of past and future and language system of their own. Thus, it is experimentally proved that few animals, if not all, are capable of being considered as persons, to become qualified to have rights.

Now the question that should be taken into consideration is — what kind of persons can have rights and under what conditions of possession and dispossession?

If it is argued that beings who are morally autonomous and who can make a choice between actions can be qualified as persons, then the argument will exclude not only non-human animals but also the insane and mentally retarded people with children, who are not autonomous beings and cannot think on their own. This implies that there are humans who cannot be considered as qualified persons, but they still enjoy the special privileges just like persons. Carl Cohen (1998:831) criticizing the view that animals have rights, argues that humans are of such a kind that they may be the subject of experiments only with their voluntary consent. The choices they make freely must be respected. Animals are of such a kind that it is impossible for them, in principle, to give or withhold voluntary consent or to make a moral choice. What humans retain when disabled, animals have never had. Nevertheless, even if animals never had rights, it is difficult to understand how disabled humans, even without being able to make a choice, can retain his rights. Further, when we don't harm even the non persons of our own species is it morally justifiable on our part to kill the non-human animals? As we protect the lives of the non-persons of our own species should we not do the same for non-persons of other species also? This, further, raises the ethical questions such as; is person-hood the only criterion to live on the earth? Is personhood a criterion for not being killed?

And also, as the above discussion exposes the few difficulties regarding person-hood being the special privilege of humans, if it is wrong to kill a person when we can avoid doing so, and there is real doubt about whether a being we are thinking of killing is a person, then should we not give that being benefit of doubt?

Now the problem, further, is whether to treat non-human animals also as having the same rights as that of humans. Whether it is Contractarians or Kantians both believe, since animals did not contract or do not belong to the moral community they have no rights. Of course, it is true that animals have no rights and in this sense they are unequal with the humans. However, the argument is, since the rights to which the Contractarians or Kantians are referring are invented by humans for the smooth running of the society and since they are invented to control the behaviour of humans over humans — only humans can hold rights and only on humans are these rights applicable. Now the question is — what right humans have over the non-humans? Of course, humans might be endowed with rationality and privileged birth from God and may possess complicated thought and language structure — however, does that make life of the non-human animals worthless and less significant? In other words, since the rights of the humans are applicable only on humans, how can right of treating animals like things by humans be justified? Aren't there any limitations to the rights of the humans?

Further, when we are talking about animal rights we are not referring to political, social and legal rights of the human world, rather we are referring to the basic right of the natural world as well as to the moral right of the artificial world. The norms which constitute or back up animal rights are moral norms. Thus, animal rights can exist, if at all, only if substantive moral norms in some sense exist. If we come to the natural world where the basic and the principled right of all human beings is, the right to life — all the beings, whether human or non-human, possess this right equally and at the time of any discrepancy the stronger party claims the victory. Since man is said to be strongest of all animals, when his physical and intellectual abilities taken together, he can make his natural right prevail over the other beings. However, this assumption is applicable only when the natural right, i.e., right to life of human beings come into clash with the non-human beings. In other words, human's right over non-humans is justified only in case of a clash for the right to life between them. That is, if the lives of both human and non-humans are at stake, then by following the above argument, the right of the humans should sustain over that of non-humans. However, in many instances where non-humans are killed by the humans, there is no stake for the human life.

Though, it is true that animals have no moral rights over humans, at least from the point of view of the humans, who consider themselves to be the superior species and moral custodians, is it morally justifiable to treat non-human animals as mere inanimate things. The following facts about the animals make them consider as morally significant beings, if not as moral agents or right-holders.

1. Pleasure and pain are equally applicable to animals.
2. The very justification of humans for using animals in experiments shows that they are similar to humans in crucial respects.

3. The very fact that we treat few humans, such as orphans, children, handicaps and mentally retarded people, with special care under protection, makes us to give minimum respect to the basic rights of animals. For, apes, monkeys, dogs and even mice and rats are more intelligent, more aware of what is happening to them and more sensitive to pain than the above mentioned non-persons of the human species.
4. Irrespective of species, sex, race and religion, all living beings have inherent value. It is not the person-hood, rather the inherent value of life that must be taken notice in arguing for animals. All beings have inherent value, all possess it equally and all have an equal right to be treated with respect, to be treated in ways that do not reduce them to the status of things, as if they existed as resources of others.

Finally, the point is not whether animals are moral agents/ beings. But, rather, since we are moral agents — is it right on our part to inflict pain or to take away not only the right, but the life of a being which is non-human.

Conclusion

To recall, the use of animals by humans may be categorized into at least five headings : 1. Food, 2. Research, 3. Entertainment, 4. Commercial purpose, 5. Superstitious believes. Almost all kinds of the violation of animal rights could be classified into any one of the above mentioned list. However, many people, if not all, including few of those who argue against animal rights, will accept that using animals for entertainment, commercial purpose and superstitious believes is wrong. Ill-treatment of the animals on the name of training to give entertainment in circus and movies is truly condemnable. Killing animals in order to sell their skin and other parts of body is no doubt most inhuman. Sacrificing animals for superstitious believes is highly repugnable. The people who support the animals sacrifice argue that the animal that is sacrificed will go to heaven. In this connection it is interesting to note that Carvakas, one of the oldest materialistic and heterodox schools of India, argued against animal sacrifice by saying that, if it is true that the animal sacrificed will go to heaven, then why not the sacrificer sacrifice his own father or grand-father, so that they can reach heaven safely. Nevertheless, coming back to the point, many people accept these three uses of animals by humans as most rejectable. However, the problem comes with the first two uses of animals, food and research, both of which are regarded to be necessary for the sustenance of the human race. One feeds millions of people and another protects people from innumerable diseases.

Use of animals for food is probably the most widespread form of animal use. Peter Singer (1993:62), while arguing that animal flesh is a luxury rather than a necessity, brings out few interesting points to our notice:

1. The overwhelming weight of medical evidence indicates that animal flesh is not necessary for good health or longevity.
2. Nor is animal production in industrialized societies an efficient way of producing food, since most of the animals consumed have been fattened on grains and other food that we could have eaten directly. When we feed these grains to animals, only about 10 per cent of the nutritional value remains as meat for human consumption. According to singer animals are treated like machines that convert fodder into flesh and people consume it because they like it.

These facts show that using animals for food cannot be justified on either health ground or on the ground that vegetarian food cannot support the whole population on earth.

The justification given for using animals in experiments is that they will reveal valuable insights about animals. They help to reduce the human suffering. Cohen (1998:834) argues that, the sum of the benefits of animal use is utterly beyond quantification. "The elimination of horrible diseases, the increase of longevity, the avoidance of great pain, the saving of lives and the improvement of quality of life achieved through the use of animals in research, is so incalculably great that to refrain from using animals in biomedical research is, on utilitarian grounds, morally wrong."

However, can we justify the tests like Draize test and LD 50 test. Many companies test new shampoos and cosmetics on rabbits. They subject rabbits to a test called Draize test, in which concentrated solutions of the cosmetics are dripped into the eyes of rabbits. Another inhuman test that is performed on animals is LD 50. Food additives, including artificial colourings and perspectives are tested by a test designed to find the lethal dose or the level of consumption. Though few experiments may really be necessary for the life of humans, can this kind of tests be justified on the name of improving the quality of life – is really a difficult question to answer.

Our natural rights are restricted so far as not to harm the ecological balance and the non-human beings in the world. Our duties are extended not only to serve and respect our own species but also we have a duty towards non-human animals which have no voice. We have to leave them, if not help them, on their own to lead a free life?

In the natural world, instead of rights, humans, as one of the many species, have duties towards nature in general and non-human animals in specific. These duties I call the rights of the animals.

When we are talking about ethical treatment of animals we are not talking in terms of either Aristotelian or Contractarian ethics or Kantian ethics. Rather the argument for animal rights rests on a broader perspective and framework than the posited by the philosophical traditions. The framework must go beyond the human artificial world and expand to the natural world where man is only one among the many species. It may be true that he may be more privileged than other species. However, he should use this privilege given by God or nature for sustenance and development of the natural world. He should act as a protector of ecological balance rather than the destroyer of the natural world. Numbers of species have extinguished and any more are getting extinguished because of man's artificial interference into the natural world by alienating himself from nature. Numbers of species which are created by nature to help man are no more now. If this continues the ecological balance will get disturbed and man can become the destroyer of his own fate.

NOTES

Bentham, J. *Introduction to the Principles of Morals and Legislation.* New York Hafner Publishers. 1749.

Cohen, Carl. "The case for the use of animals in Biomedical research" in *Ethics, History, Theory and Contemporary Issues,* eds. Steven M. Cohn and Peter Markie, New York: Oxford University Publications.

Kant, I. *Fundamental Principles of the Metaphysic of Morals.* New York. Liberal Arts Press. 1949.

Regan, T. *The Case for Animal Rights.* Berkeley. University of California Press. 1983.

Routledge Encyclopedia of Philosophy.

Singer, P. *Practical Ethics.* Cambridge. Cambridge University Press. 1993.

Singer, P. *Animal Liberation.* New York. Avon Books. 1975.

Chapter 13

Morality of Human Sexuality

M.P. Chaurasia

Aspects, Meaning and Purposes of Human Sexuality

Sex is an essential phenomenon, not only of human beings but also of animals and insects. But sexual relationships of animals are not the *subject matter* of ethics, because animals are considered to be irrational and their sexual activities do not affect others. But so far human beings, sexual activities come under the purview of moral consideration, because their actions may go to affect other individual's social life. The human sexual activity has three-fold meaning and purposes, e.g., procreation, pleasure and an expression of love for other individuals. These are not mutually exclusive because, very often it can be limited to only one of these purposes. The general opinion concerning the human sexuality from the very dawn of the civilization (especially from the religious point of view), is procreation. From the *psychological point* of view, it is the deepest and most intimate expression of the love of man for one another. But it should never be taken to mean that all love is sexual activity only. Apart from sexual activity, love may also be possible in many cases. For example, love between brother and sister, mother and son, father and son or daughter does not consist of sex-activity. Though Foucault and other post-modern thinkers have mentioned incestuous love but that is exception. (Levistrauss, "Do dual Organisations existing", in *Structural Anthropology*, pp.123-63, for wide discussion also see Jacques Lacan, "And this is why Sexuality is always a play of Masks and disguises" in *Fifty Key Contemporary Thinkers*, Routledge, New York, 1994, p. 69) But whenever there is the question of a meaningful love, it implies sexual activity. Sexual love is deeper than all other forms of love, as it is a new kind of experience full of thrills and sensations, which were never experienced before such relationship adds a rich dimension to the life of person concerned which is not possible in other kind of love. Sexuality (sexual relations) means conjugation or co-habitation between the opposite sexes.

In our preliminary society, even in modern society, some people think that the human sexuality implies procreation, taking it as not a very important aspect of human relationships of human life. In Islamic culture, even today and in ancient Hindu culture too, sexual activity is highly protected and prohibited phenomenon of human life. In Islamic nations, even today, capital punishment is imposed for pre-*nikah* cohabitation. In ancient Indian culture too, many laws were made to stop such activity. Generally the members of our conservative society do not consider love aspect of sex rather they ignore this aspect. Still today many persons think of sex as a dirty evil. If we analyse the spirit of eighteenth and nineteenth centuries laws of our country, we shall find an attitude of such kind. In that era, all kinds of private sexual activity between even consenting adults were forbidden, for this or that reason. In our country during middle age, if a wife has sexual relationship with any person other than her husband, she was liable to be punished bitterly. But these days such laws are not prevalent in our society. Latest development in this context is the finding of Master and Johnson (*Human Sexual Response*, Boston: Little Brown, 1966) According to them, these laws reflected a view of human sexual activity, which does not square with studies made in the twentieth century. The scope of human sexuality is very limited and it is also a dissatisfied relation, because people are given to such upbringing that they are strongly influenced by the taboos established by their ancestors against meaningful sexual relations, set-up and sanctioned by the concerning society. So we may say that the expression of love aspect of human sexual activity is no less important than procreation and it should be emphasized more than in the past, for the sake of pleasure.

Our traditional society always thinks of sexual activity either in terms of procreation aspect or as a necessary evil. They had emphasized it under *biological urge* felt by man and not by woman, because it is man who seeks satisfaction by cohabitation. On the other side the supporters of complete freedom in sexual matters usually insist the pleasure aspect and the right of individuals to enjoy such pleasure. In this context there is also a moderate view according to which procreation and pleasure are the essential aspects of sexuality but we cannot and should not ignore the importance of its love aspect. While the supporters of free-sex accept only the love aspect in sexual activity.

Now we should distinguish the factors that are responsible to make a difference between public aspect and private aspect of human sexuality. The public aspect of sex means the way in which sex matters affect others. And from this point of view, the basic controlling principles of morality are life, goodness and justice. While the private aspect is related with sexual relations between consenting adults and the basic governing principles in this regard are those of goodness, justice, freedom and honesty. Here, we should distinguish between two kinds of actions that involve in human sexuality: those that have such a harmful effect on people other than involved in this activity and so they should be prohibited by moral rules or law, and those which affect only the participants must be overruled for the sake of people concerned. The most vital question in this regard is whether we should restrict such activity or allow a great deal of sexual freedom?

As I feel, there are a few sexual activities which should be morally condemned. Those activities are also highly offensive from the point of view of law of the land. Any sexual activity which is performed against the will of the either party is wholly wrong. From this angle, rape, child molestation and sadism are performed against the will of the victims. Such sexual acts immediately affect the public or individual in a unique way. These three sexual acts badly harm the life of concerning people upon which such actions are performed. In certain such cases, insanity and even death of the people occurs. We should always condemn such sexual activity. We do not have knowledge of that moral principle under which certain people perform such heinous acts like rape, molestation and sadism. But almost all people agree that these acts are highly immoral and should be stopped by any means. There are a few other sexual activities which need to be checked up, these are pornography, homosexuality, sex outside marriage (premarital and extramarital sex), adultery, masturbation and perverted sexual activity. But all people do not have the same moral views regarding these activities as all have in case of rape, molestation and sadism.

The Views against Sexual Freedom

As per recent trend, perhaps, people who believe in traditional values are considered conservative. They consider moral value as 'absolute' and think that sexual freedom is a violation of this value, which is part and parcel of our Indo-Aryan heritage. Our traditional concept of social order allows only heterosexual sex, because only this kind of sexuality is morally permissible. They also suggest the method of cohabitation. According to the religious faith, sexual acts should be performed in natural way, i.e., man should hold woman from the top and woman should lie under him. According to this view sexual activity should take place only between legally married couple. Here 'legally married' means marriage between one man and one woman. Again, the conjugally allied partners should cohabit not for the sake of pleasure or love but only to produce children. Besides this sexual activity all other forms of sexual acts are the violations of the traditional moral teachings, because polygamy, sex-outside of marriage, homosexuality and perverted sexual activity, tend to destroy the peace and pleasure of family and social life. Lastly, these practices destroy the sanctity of the above institutions.

If pornography, molestation and 'perverted' sexual activity are allowed, then immature children and innocent people may also get involved in these activities. Consequently there will be an increase in rapes, child molestation and sadism. All these activities will be performed on unwilling victims. If sexual freedom is allowed, we cannot stop these activities and would result into sexual murders. Pornography on T.V., Internet, in newspapers and films inflames the sexual appetites or desires of people, especially the adolescent youth so much that they try to find outlets for these appetites somehow and resort to these unacceptable means. If more sexual freedom is allowed, it would undermine our social values. All the good and decent things from the society, such as family, respect for marriage, love without lust, regard for men and women and respect for children would vanish. If we glance over the taste of the public, we find that people easily accept heterosexual relationships, monogamous marriages and sexual activity within a marriage institution, while they do not easily accept homosexual relationships, polygamous marriages and sexual activity outside marriage institution.

Recent research also proves that pornography in all forms is harmful for the society. Julia Heman, the director of *the Kinly Institute for Research in Sex, Gender and Reproduction*, in a seminar organized at Santa Fay on "The Future of Sex" shows much anxiety over the increase of solitary sexual activity, because it is imaginary. The sexual activity sponsored by Internet through Cyber Cafe, damage the sex life of individuals as it provokes sexual activity more and more without partner. If people involve themselves more and more in solitary and imaginary sexual activity, actual sex-life would not be required at all. Cyber sex, on the force of vigour and zest of Viagra and other medicines, can attract people toward itself, but such activity always ends in a kind of deep depression, because real life cannot defeat the imagination. According to Heman, if our youths learn sexuality through such a manner, then what will be the fate of real conjugal life that happens in pure solitude in contact with one's bed partner at night? All claims made by the medicine companies are false. In the same way Prof. John Gegnon of the State University of New York claims that medicine to increase the power of retention also deforms the nature of original sex life and increase the problem of solitary sex day-by-day. These medicines separate original sex couples more than to congregate them. Again, sex served by music, magazines, T.V., films and Cyber Cafe are pushing children towards sexuality in their early ages. According to Jen Brown of North Carrolina University, this is first time that we see that for the sake of money, children are also included in sex-shows. Such activity increase at the rate of 2.2 per cent children in sex activity per year. [*Hindustan Dainik* Patna 2006, p.16] After seeing the above consequences, nobody can support the view of sexual-freedom.

Pro-Sex Freedom

Supporters of individual freedom argue that people ought to have the freedom to do what they like to do, because they are consenting adults provided, they do not harm physically or directly the other members of the society by their actions. If they do not commit rape, or molest children or perform sadistic acts on unwilling victims then why society would have any complaint against their sexual freedom? They should be provided complete freedom in the field of sex to do what they like to do with consenting adults even in or outside marriage. Society have no right to forbid without finding something wrong to as long as their actions do not harm other people.

Undoubtedly traditional morality in the field of sex, once upon a time has served the society in many ways, but such morality cannot be and should not be regarded absolute, as nothing is absolute in ethics. All our traditions are based on archaic views of the biological and psychological make up of human beings — views, which are turned down by the researches of twenty first century in the field of sciences and social sciences. Now-a-days we know more about sex than our ancestors and have searched out a wider and open expression of love and pleasure, which are most important factors of human life. We do not have any clear and distinct indication in a religious book that God and nature have prescribed such and such conduct in sexuality except certain prohibitions, which one may obey or disobey. They do consider marriage as sacrament rather a contract made on a piece of paper and, they insist, that there is evidence that the sex which takes place outside marriage is as meaningful as that which takes place within his institution. According to them sex between homosexual, polygamous relationships or in a monogamous marriage is alike and thc same. Every individual is different and unique, their feelings and desires must vary from one person to another. Therefore, they ought to be allowed the complete freedom of sexual expression as long as they do not harm others.

The proponents of sexual freedom further argue that there is no strong evidence which suggests that if sexual freedom is granted then there is a violation in the areas of rape, incest and sadism. For example, in Denmark pornography has been made completely legal and there it is freely available, but there is a decrease in the rate of sexual crime, child molestation and forced sadism. Supporters of sexual freedom conceive pornography as a force that relieves sexual tensions and eliminates the need for harmful sexual activities. If for some time it is accepted that such freedom cause sexual murder, then what our laws do? There are certain laws to stop such crime and we have no complaints against these laws. Then why sexual freedom should be restricted or refrained.

To say that sexual freedom is against public taste, is wrong because this cannot be a strong reason to censor the freedom of sex. In real sense, it is simply a violation of customs and manners than a disregard for morality. If we do not violate the principle of justice in any sense, because offensiveness to public taste does not mean the violation of justice while bodily harm or sex-murder is not only unethical but also a crime. We do not say that public taste should not be considered. If we are always careful to the feelings and rights of others, and, we do not compel others to participate in our activities, we never perform sexual activities in an open place, then our actions would not harm others? Therefore, if we enjoy sexual freedom with consenting adults among ourselves, society should not raise a hue and cry?

Sex Within and Outside Marriage

Now, we shall consider mainly monogamous marriage type sex, polygamous marriage type sex, sex outside marriage and premarital sex. The first objection against premarital sexuality is that it will destroy the high tradition and sanctity of marriage institution of our society. Generally all conservative societies based on different religions very rigidly follow such values. According to the tradition, sex should be reserved till marriage and it can be allowed only to produce children and for no other purposes. Again it should be confined within heterosexual monogamous marriage only. And only such sexuality should be prolonged in our society. If premarital sex is allowed it will discourage the special and holy status of monogamous marriage institution. Premarital sex also encourages an inflated view of sex as the most important aspect of marriage, thereby further eroding one of our best social institutions. Sexuality is an inseparable part of marriage institution and if it is available without marriage, then why will people marry? And in this way our social life will be scattered into pieces.

Supporters of premarital sex are of the view that our traditions gradually change with changing modes of scientific researches, technological developments and rapidly changing life styles. The institution of family is not the same as in the sixteenth century. It is now more mobile and flexible in accordance with the modern culture. Certainly some bad changes have come in our culture, but modern men need many alternatives of life styles and premarital sex is one of them, because it provokes freedom and individuality. In traditional society, marriage meant a dictator husband and his slave wife who are free to make illegal relation with other woman. Many premarital sex relations have converted into marriages. In premarital sex there is no scope for promiscuity, while its several examples are found in married pairs. So far the concept of guilt complex is concerned, it is matter for those who do it. If somehow woman becomes pregnant, there are several ways to get relief from pregnancy and if there is no way, marriages are the last solution. The proponents also plead that they use contraception regularly, so there is no fear of pregnancy.

The strongest argument in this context of the proponents is to gain experience and compatibility in the field of sex. In our society, people think that sexual activity is a natural ability that one can easily acquire after marriage but the fact is not so, because sexual relationship is not merely a biological coupling. It is a highly complex matter and needs a great deal of knowledge and ability. These abilities do not come naturally because these need a hard patience to acquire, especially in a culture like ours where sex is repressed for a long time. If premarital sex is allowed, youth will evaluate themselves whether they are sexually able for marriages or not, as they have already acquired more experience and compatibility. Learning through experience is one thing, and to do simply on the basis of hearing is another thing. Through experience people realized themselves what types of relationships they like and with what type of person they can adjust. In this way if they discover that they are not compatible, they separate themselves friendly.

The great advantage of premarital sexuality is to gain more and more pleasure as both the partners have no responsibility. So by allowing premarital sex, sexual pleasure can be enjoyed freely to the extent individual wishes without permanent commitment. So this should be left for those who like it. This is purely private matter and so it should be left to the discretion of free consenting adults. The premarital sexuality is not a new event in our society. In the *Mahabharata,* the case of Kunti and in the *Ramayana*, the request of Surpanakha to Laxman is the kind of premarital sex. Even today if we glance over the way of life of a remote village, we shall find that there are also the cases of premarital sex. T.V. and Media propagate sexuality on such a high level that ebullience of sexuality has come on the surface. We are unable to stop this ebullition. So this matter should be left on the free choices of the people.

Now we shall consider the marriage type sex which means, in many cases permanent sexual relationships though it has also some overlapping. Such overlapping may be considered as extramarital relationships that occur among married couples. The purposes of marriage are at least three: procreation, love for one another and pleasure. Almost all religions of the world support this view except in few cases in Islam. But those who do not have faith in religion they never care of such belief. If the chief aim of sexuality is a deep and close expression of love, and if procreation is only secondary then how we can morally blame homosexuality as it does produce nothing. The traditional people criticize homosexuality because it is unnatural and does not produce children like heterosexuality. Some people cast aside homosexuality saying that it is the activity of abnormal man. But individuals who have engaged themselves in such activities, do not accept the blame of abnormality. They claim that they are as good a moral person as anybody can be. They look differently, because they have selected a separate sexual life style.

Another kind of extramarital sexual relationship is adultery. We can underline many kinds of sexual relationship under this title, e.g., sexual relations outside of marriage, contract agreement or relationship. Adultery means the voluntary engaging in sexual relation with someone other than one's married partner. Such kind of relationship is an unfaithful action in the marriage relationship, especially in its sexual aspects and so it is considered by all as immoral. But we have no criteria to decide whether such action is moral or immoral.

In our society many marriages do not seem what actually they are, because one or both partners may not relate well with each other at any level. This means they are dissatisfied even on sexual level also and so they look for other human relationship that fulfil them in ways their own marriage relationship will not. Whenever the marriage relationship is an unhappy one, people are compelled to engage in adultery with the persons who make them happy separately. Or they both gain more pleasure from the new relationships than their original marriage. In such a relation people generally begin the adultery relation and if per chance of eventuality worry about its consequence later on. Sometimes innocent wife becomes the victim of such relationship and she commits suicide to leave the children in destitution.

So adultery is a direct violation of the most sacred and intimate human contract into which people generally enter by their own will. On the eve of marriage general men and women make a contract to live together as husband and wife and remain faithful to one another. If they both commit or one of them commits adultery, it involves lying, cheating and infidelity on the part of one's marriage partner or another and these actions are immoral in any ethical system. In some cases both wife and husband are ready to consent adultery, for example, in case of exchange of wives they are abusing the marriage institution. If they want such freedom, they should not marry at all. But the only merit of such activities in exchange of wives is that both the partners know the truth and they agree to enjoy the change. So there is no question of dishonesty.

There are several arguments in favour of adultery. First of all people are of the view that individuals ought to be free to do what they want to do in terms of their own private sex lives and to what extent they cheat their partner, are their personal matter, not of the society. Basically people involved in such activity are unaware of the consequence. When adultery is discovered, bad result occurs. In another argument adulterers say that if they are wise enough and can avert breaking up their family then what is bad with these activities? Some persons who support adultery argue that in one way we save our family and children too, because it provides a means through which unsatisfied spouses satisfy their lusts. Wives, husbands and children continue to have social and economic security and adulterous spouses additionally enjoy a happy sex life. If the affair is not disclosed for a long time, what is bad with adultery? In the same way, exchange of wives is a different sexual life style, and as long as adult couples freely consent to such activity, no harm is done to any one. These all are private matters and society should never intervene in any way.

Now we should consider the ethical principles involved in sexuality. Undoubtedly Value of Life Principle is not involved in private sexuality, as it is based on adult consent. But any case which is life threatening must be considered immoral. The

Principles of Goodness is essentially involved in this activity, as sexual activity should cause pleasure and avoid pain. So it should be performed for excellence, should encourage harmony among all concerned. People who indulge in this play should make a strong attempt to be honest and tell the truth in all aspects of human relationship. Further in matters of private sexuality, individual freedom should be the guiding principle as long as the rights of the persons directly involve in this relationship. All kinds of rapes, child molestation and sadism are considered wholly immoral. All sexual activities performed between the consenting adults are moral as long as it cannot harm others.

Chapter 14

Bioethics and the Buddha

Angraj Chaudhary

Bioethics means the ethics of medical and biological research. Researchers in these fields have made a quantum leap in the present century. Medical researchers are making various researches to discover medicines for different kinds of diseases. Some of the medicines discovered indeed have miraculous effects. But these medicines are discovered by making experiments on mice, guinea pigs, cows and horses. Researchers test different kinds of medicine on them and ascertain the suitability or otherwise of medicines for mankind. During these experiments the innocent and mute animals suffer severe pains and even die during the process. The question is — Is it ethically justified to make experiments on the mute and innocent animals, cause them severe pain and even cause their death? The answer to this question can partly be found in another question— Can the discovered medicines be directly experimented on human beings. This is what some of the scientists of Hopkins Institute in collaboration with some Indian scientists did recently and with what result. They are feeling a lot of guilt conscience.

There are some thinkers and social workers, who are dead against making experiments on animals because in the process a lot of injury and pain is inflicted on them. This, according to them, is cruelty towards animals and highly unethical. But will they allow scientists to experiment discovered medicines directly on man? And what would the Buddha have to say about it?

Had the Buddha been alive today, could he have shut his eyes to these cruel acts? Could he have allowed researchers to perpetrate such horrible crimes on mute animals? Before answering these questions one would like to put two counter questions. If one of the disciples of the Buddha were to suffer from a disease and the doctor prescribed such medicines as are discovered in the way described above, could he have forbidden his disciple to take such medicines? And could he have allowed scientists to experiment the discovered medicines directly on human beings and risk their lives?

To my mind, as the Buddha considered man's life very valuable, perhaps more valuable than the lives of other creatures in the world, and as his philosophy is exclusively humanitarian, geared to the spiritual development of man besides solving other problems of life, he would have definitely cared more for their physical and mental health.

We know that the Buddha regarded man as the greatest of all beings. To be born as man is the highest advantage, specially from the spiritual point of view, because it is man who can become a Buddha, it is he who can practise *Dhamma* and attain *nirvana*. This view of the Buddha is corroborated by what he says in the *Buddhavamsa—Manussattam liṅga sampatti Satthāram dassanam* etc. Out of the eight chief conditions, which are necessary for attaining Buddhahood, to be born as man is the first important condition. The other conditions follow from this. It is man who can attain *vijja (paññā)* and *caraṇa (sila and samādhi)—Vijjā carana sampanno, so settho devamānuseti*, other beings can not. So in the scale of values, man occupies the highest place.

The second point the Buddha makes is that in order to walk on the Noble Eightfold Path one must have fairly good health. It is only healthy people free from diseases who can perform the uphill task of treading on the Noble Eightfold Path. *Śarīramadyam khalu dharma sādhamam.* To begin with a healthy body is the primary requisite for practising religion.

So man's life being valuable, must, on all accounts, be saved. Medical researchers who make experiments on animals in order to discover suitable and efficacious medicines for mankind cannot be ethically blamed because, in the first place, their intention is not to take their life. Killing or murder is said to be committed when five conditions are fulfilled, viz., there must be a being to be killed, there must be a killer, it must be his intention to kill, he must have a weapon to kill (he can use his hands and legs as weapons) and when the act of killing is actually committed. We also know that many bacteria are killed when we breathe in and breathe out but we commit no murder as our intention is not to kill them.

And, in the second place, the medicines they discover save precious human lives. In short, the *akusala kamma* they do (if at all they do it) is more than compensated by the (*kusala kamma*) they do. Just as a ball of iron immediately sinks into the sea but a ship made of tonnes of iron does not, so the *kusala kamma* done in discovering medicines to save precious human lives acts as a ship which can carry several balls of iron symbolising *akusala kamma* without sinking. Researchers make experiments without having the intention to kill the animals they experiment on. So their intention being pure they are not ethically blameworthy and the harm that they do is more than compensated by the good that they do. Besides, *kamma visaya* is the subject of the Buddha, it is *acintanya* for us. We never know in what proportion and in what way we get the results of the *kammas* we do.

Buddha's great concern was to root out the cause of suffering and annihilate it. In order to do so, he prescribed a way for purifying mind from pollutants like cravings and aversions—the cause of suffering. But although he prescribed a way alright he did not make it binding for all to walk upon it. He was not a theoretical philosopher like many others who only think about a problem intellectually. He was a realist. He knew very well the different capacities of individuals and, therefore, he did not expect all to follow what he prescribed . Of course, as he established an order of monks who had left home for leading a homeless life in order to attain *nibbāna*, (*amata, deathlessness*), he prescribed the great mass of rules for its members with a view to guiding them in such a way that they could live a monastic life smoothly without violating the ethical codes of conduct which are the backbone of leading a spiritual life. So he made the great mass of *Vinayic* rules binding for them. He prescribed in detail the do's and dont's for monks and nuns. What kinds of shoes and sandals the monks might wear and whether they should make use of animals' skin or hides have been discussed in detail. It is clear from the *Vinaya Patrika* that whatever the Buddha prescribed and what he objected to are based on sound reason. Nothing that he said, prescribed or not allowed is arbitrary. He was not rigid, but he was always open to conviction and adapted himself to the changed circumstances. He did not make it compulsory for a Sona Kolivisa who was delicately nurtured to go without a sandal nor did he ask a monk with corns in his feet to negotiate the road without shoes, nor did he ask the monks to make use of animals' skins when he did not consider them necessary. Of course, his intention was not to take life, however, infinitesimal. So he did not allow monks to use animals' hides, but when he saw it was necessary for monks living in the border country where, perhaps, the winter was not kind he prescribed, animals' hides for them to keep themselves from inclement weather. Wooden shoes were objected to because monks wearing them might slip on insects and kill them besides disturbing the monks who were meditating.

It is true one of the most important five ethical precepts is to abstain from killing, but it must be remembered that he did not prescribe it for all. When soldiers fight in the war in order to defend their country from enemies, they are bound to kill and the Buddha considered it the bounden duty of the soldiers to fight and kill. That is why when he came to know that the king's soldiers stealthily entered the order and some monks ordained them as monks, the Buddha admonished such monks and did not allow such soldiers to be ordained. He knew that there are different duties to be performed by different persons and performing different duties is essential for making a society stable and smooth going. He did not confuse worldly obligations with spiritual ones, So he did not interfere in others' affairs. But personally he liked to walk on the Noble Eightfold Path, observe *sila*, practice *samādhi* and attain *paññā* to know the true nature of reality and realizing at the experiential level the transitory and fleeting nature of worldly objects develop non-attachment (*nirveda*) to them and break the strong bonds that bind one to the wheel of life and death. He kept on giving this message to all and sundry, but never made it binding for all. Of course, he hoped his message was driven home to many so that they could realize the sweeter and higher values of life and being inspired by their conviction they could walk on the path of virtue. It is true he was greatly concerned with spiritual life, but he did not lose sight of the material life and material well-being here and now.

If we read the section on medicines in the *Mahāvagga*, it will soon be amply clear that the Buddha was not rigid and whatever he prescribed as medicines he did not do it arbitrarily. In the beginning when he prescribed five medicines such as ghee, fresh butter, oil, honey and molasses to monks and nuns he prescribed them knowing full well that they are medicines and are also agreed upon as medicines". This phrase is very important because the Buddha accepted those as medicines, which people regarded as medicines. People must have accepted them as medicines after seeing their efficacy in curing diseases and for determining their efficacious nature some sort of experiments must have gone on even in those days and, may be, they were experimented on animals and birds. He did not bother his head to know how they were procured, by killing animals or by any other means. If ill monks had need of tallows as medicines he allowed them. "I allow you monks, to make use of tallows as medicines by using them with oil: tallow from bears, tallow from fish, tallow from alligators, tallow from swine, tallow from donkeys..." (*The Book of the Discipline*, Vol 4; pp. 270-271). Didn't the Buddha know that the tallows are got from killing these animals? On another occasion when he came to know that a monk who had a non-human affliction got cured when he ate raw flesh and drank raw blood of a swine in a swine's slaughter-place, he allowed other monks suffering from it to take it. "I allow, monks, when one has a non-human affliction, raw flesh and raw blood" (*ibid.*, p. 274). Didn't he know that raw flesh and raw blood of a swine can be obtained only by killing swine?

The Buddha was able to make a distinction between what is necessary and life saving and what is not. Therefore, he did not allow monks to wear shoes of palmyra palm leaves, because when they are cut, they wither and die. But he did allow them to use roots of turmeric, ginger, orris root, white orris root, garlic, black hellebore, khus-khus, nut grass or whatever other roots there are that are medicines, knowing full well that when their roots are dug up, they will die.

In the light of what has been said above the Buddha would have allowed such medicines as are available in the market, although they are procured from animals which suffer severe pain and even die. But this is another question whether the Buddha, if asked for permission, would have allowed scientists to inflict so much pain on innocent animals to discover medicines?

We know he did not allow a monk to treat patients but he did not make it ethically binding for all, who can, not to make researches in medicine and discover life saving medicines. After all, the Buddha did not hesitate in taking the services of *Jivaka Komārabhacca*, whose fame as a great surgeon had spread far and wide and who 'having cut open the skin of his (a merchant of Rajgir) head, having opened a suture in the skull' drew out two living creatures and cured the disease of his head'. The Buddha knew it but he did not regard him as a violator of the first ethical principle although the two creatures he had drawn out from the merchant's head must have perished soon.

Chapter 15

Buddha's View on Transplantation of Human Organs

Angraj Chaudhary

What would have been the view of the Buddha on transplantation of human organ, had he lived now? This is a very intriguing question but a very relevant one. Any ethics or ethical precept in order to be universal, has to stoutly face the challenges of changing times and not become irrelevant. We have to examine here whether Buddha's ethical precepts stand the test of the time.

It is true that the Buddha does not say anything directly on transplantation of human organ. How could he do so? There came no occasion in his life when he was faced with such a problem. Neither there was so much of biomedical research in his time, nor could the doctors of his time ever think of replacing any damaged human organs by another human organ. The well-known doctor Jivaka – Buddha's personal physician could perform miraculous surgery[1] but there is no reference to his transplanting human organ. This is a contribution of modern science and modern biomedical research.

If a man is suffering from a damaged kidney or if both of his kidneys are damaged and there is no hope of his survival, the doctor can ensure his survival today by transplanting one or both of his kidneys. We know that each one of us has two kidneys, so if we agree to donate one kidney, we can save the life of a man whose both kidneys are damaged.

I do not think the Buddha could ever have raised any objection to the transplantation of human organs, if by doing so a precious human life could be saved. If a man can live with one kidney, donate the other to one whose both kidneys are damaged, it is well and good, because by donating one of his kidneys, he saves a precious human life. Not only does he earn merit by doing so, but also he helps other human being to see some more springs in this world and do some more *kusala kamma*.

We know that the tradition of donating organs or limbs is very ancient in India. In the hoary past we hear of the great sage Dadhici donating his bone to gods with which they could vanquish the Asuras. At other time we hear of King Sivi who, while he was a Bodhisattva, gave his eyes to a blind man.

But the Buddha definitely would have strongly objected to the racket of supplying kidneys to the needy ones for fabulous money by playing fraud on the person from whom they are taken. This racket has become rampant in modern times particularly in our country.

When the question of the transplantation of kidney comes, there are three possibilities. Either some near and dear ones of the person whose both kidneys become non functional donates one of his or her kidney and saves his life or the ailing person buys the kidney from someone who willingly sells it for money. There is nothing unethical in these two cases. The donor by donating the kidney saves the life of other, without doing harm to his or her life. If under good medical care, experts perform such operation as taking out one kidney from one and transplanting it on the other, both lives can be saved. Many persons have undergone such operations and many lives have been saved.

There are persons, as has been said above, who have the volition to donate their organs to save the lives of their near and dear ones and even to save the lives of other human beings. Recently I heard a news on the B.B.C. about a daughter making up her mind to donate a kidney as a Christmas gift and save the life of her father who has been on dialysis for seven long years. Isn't this an excellent and sublime Christmas gift? Had the Buddha been living today he would have definitely said, sādhu, sādhu (very well, very well).

There is nothing unethical in somebody selling his or her kidney for money. If he or she agrees to sell his or her kidney for money what is unethical about it? In fact, the donee would ever remain grateful to him or her although he has bought it from him or her for money.

But there are cases where doctors take a patient to OT to operate, say, on his appendix and while he is under the influence of anesthesia his kidney is taken out for sale at a fantastic price in the market. The patient does not know that without his consent, one of his kidneys has been removed. This is highly unethical. This is highly unethical in two ways. The patient's kidney is removed without his consent and the life saved may be that of a criminal or a very bad person from whom no good is expected. In fact, if he survives, he may do more harm to the people and society with his lengthened life. Thus the doctor removing the kidney of a patient who was to be operated on appendix commits twofold crime. He removes the kidney of a patient without his consent and inflicts a great psychological injury to him. Besides, being psychologically scared about his physical health, he loses faith in his doctor so much so that he would never like to entrust himself to any other doctor and hazard his other organ being removed. Once bitten he becomes twice shy. He becomes weak both physically and psychologically. Thus the doctor does incalculable damage to him who reposed great faith in him. This is against medical ethics Besides, what has the doctor gained? For a sum of money which will not last him long (for he is bound to ill spend it) he gives a new lease of life to one who perhaps does not deserve it and thus enables him to perpetrate more crimes than ever.

There is one more situation where the doctor along with a band of persons who thrive on such rackets forms a nexus and indulges in such activities on a large scale. A person, say, from Ranchi is persuaded to go to Madras for a job where he is hospitalized on some pretext or other and then he is divested of his kidney there. These racketeers get a huge sum, which they share with the doctor who deserves to be prosecuted for culpable homicide.

These are highly unethical acts and the Buddha would have never approved of them. So far as the ethics of organ transplantation is concerned there is nothing wrong in it, but the racket of taking out human organ and selling it for a fabulous price and saving the life of a rogue is highly unethical. Such acts are shorn of all human sentiments. They are not performed with noble sentiments of saving the life of an ailing person, but they are performed with an eye on money, not on merit.

What would the Buddha have said about human organ transplantation if a liver were transplanted on a person whose liver is irreparably damaged? We know that unlike kidney one has got only one liver. So if somebody's liver is removed to save another man's life, it is pure murder of that man from whom the liver is taken out. If somebody being fed up with life wants to donate his liver to one with a damaged liver, he will be taking his own life. Here also an ethical question is involved. Is it ethically good for a man to put an end to his life? There are different views on this question. The whole question of euthanasia comes up here.

Let us take another situation. Suppose biomedical researches say that the liver of a monkey can as well suit a man, will it be ethical to take out a monkey's liver and save one human life? Apparently it may sound ethically alright but its rampant use will create unbalance in nature and there will be the danger of entire ecology being disturbed and affected.

I think the Buddha would not have allowed a man, although incalculably suffering, to donate his liver and end his life and get rid of his suffering. This does not agree with his *Kamma* theory where a man has to undergo suffering in proportion to his unwholesome action (*akusala kamma*).

There is another situation. Suppose there is an accident and a man is soon to die. There is absolutely no possibility of his survival.

Then in that circumstance if his liver is extracted and transplanted on a person whose liver is damaged and thus enables him to live long, there is nothing wrong in it. This is ethical. Based on this principle other organs such as eye, etc., are now preserved in eyebanks, etc. and are transplanted on the needy persons. We find many persons like Aishawarya Rai who have expressed their wishes to donate their eyes. Long back I read an autobiographical essay by an eminent I.C.S. of Bihar. He had enjoyed the beauty of the jungles of Bihar. So he solemnly wrote in his will that his eyes be taken out after his death and be transplanted on some needy person so that 'his eyes' could be able to see the bewitching beauty of the jungles of Bihar for a longer period. There is nothing wrong in donating organs in such a way and for such a noble purpose.

Recently we read a very moving news. The family members of two persons who were declared clinically dead donated their bodies. With their various organs the doctors there could save the life of a 28 years old girl and that of a 24 years old young boy on whom their hearts were successfully transplanted. Four persons suffering from damaged kidneys got a new lease of life when their four kidneys were transplanted on them. Two persons with damaged livers had livers transplanted on them and two had their eyes transplanted on them. Thus the two clinically dead persons gave a new lease of life to ten persons. This may once again remind us of the great sage Dadhici. .

Now-a-days researchers in biomedical science are trying to prepare clones of different organs. If cloning of organs is successfully done, the damaged organs of persons can be replaced by organ transplantation technique. This is definitely going to greatly contribute to the health of the suffering people and reduce health hazards to a great extent. But cloning human beings will, perhaps, produce confusion. We know what happened to Dolly—the first ever sheep cloned. If clones are made to become more miserable, why clone human beings and multiply misery? For that matter why clone even animals and make their lives more miserable? Isn't there enough misery in the world?

But if cloning can be done from the organ of a healthy person without doing any damage to his health and if it is as functional and efficient as the original one why not have more such clones for transplantation on human beings whose particular organs are damaged?. But one has to be very cautious in this so that the cloned organ may not carry any disease. If it carries a disease then the person on whom the transplantation is done may get infected from a disease from which he never suffered previously. This will be like falling from a frying pan to fire.

We hear of another kind of organ transplantation. The heart is a very delicate organ. In case it becomes non-functioning, doctors now-a-days, think of replacing such a heart by pig's heart which is functionally exactly like a human heart. Naturally when the heart of a pig will be taken out for transplantation, the pig is bound to die. The question is how far it is ethical to take the life of one, even though an animal, and save the life of a human being? What would have been the Buddha's view on it?

It is true the implication of the first precept propounded by the Buddha is to be kind to all creatures, not to kill them and develop *metta* (loving kindness) towards all creatures of the world. But if we read between the lines of some of the passages in the *Tipitaka* and the commentarial literature, it will be clear that man according to him, occupies a higher place in the hierarchy of beings. It is a man who can become a Buddha, a *Pacceka* Buddha and an *Arhat*, animals cannot. To be born a man is one of the essential conditions of becoming a Buddha. It is said in the Buddhavamsa[2] that '*manussattaṃ*' is one of the important eight conditions for becoming a Buddha. *Manussattaṃ liṅgasampatti, hetu satthāradassanama*, etc. That man is the uppermost in the hierarchy of beings is also proved by what Buddhaghosa says in the context of *parajika* rule. If one intends to kill a ram in the night and by mistake kills his father or mother or an Arahant sitting there he commits a *pārājika*, he commits an action whose results follow immediately, without giving any interval. If he kills somebody else he commits *pārājika* but its results do not follow him immediately. But if he kills the ram there he commits a *pācittiya*.[3] The gravity of the offence depends upon who gets killed— a man or an animal. It is clear from such examples that for the Buddha man's life is more important than the life of an animal. One may say that there is a difference between man and man. A man may sincerely live a moral and virtuous life, the other may not. If one of them is to be saved with the resources available, which of the two should be saved? It is a very difficult question. Who will judge who is the better of the two and who should be saved? There are possibilities that a man living an immoral life now may begin to live a moral life in future so much so that he may surpass the first one and perform more wholesome *kammas* and accumulate more merit than the other. From this point of view both deserve to be saved.

So just as the Buddha allowed meat broth[4] to a monk whose body came to be full of bad humours, allowed the ill monks to use tallows[5] as medicine — tallow from bears, from fish, from alligators, from swine and from donkeys, knowing full well that 'tallows must have been obtained by killing those animals', so if the Buddha found that a pig's heart were going to save a human life he would allow the use of it. Of course, he would not directly say to kill a pig and get his heart, but if it is available he would not forbid it to be used. Human life is more precious than that of an animal.

We know that bacteria which are unicellular micro-organisms cause several diseases. When a man suffers from a wound with pus several hundred thousand of them are killed when the wound is operated. But that is allowed. The Buddha allowed a monk having boils a treatment with a lancet operation.[6] It is true that the Buddha never showed contempt for animals like St Paul did who said. "Does God care for an ox? but he never went to the extreme of observing non-violence like the Jains do. I think Itsing — the Chinese traveller, succinctly expresses the Buddha's view of non-violence when he says that "if man will protect each and every being, he will himself become unprotected and will have to lose his life for nothing".[7]

REFERENCES

1. (a) The son of a merchant of Benares suffered from a twist in the bowels. He could not digest even the conjey that he drank, let

alone digest the food that he ate. As a result, he became thin and emaciated and his colour became yellowish. Jivaka examined him and knowing the cause of his uneasiness he 'tied him to a post and placing his wife in front of him he cut open the skin of his stomach, drew out the twisted bowel, showed it to his wife and said to her that this was the cause of his uneasiness", straightened it, put it back again and stitched the skin of the stomach and applied an ointment. He soon became well. (*The Book of the Discipline* by I.B. Horner, p. 390)

(b) Jivaka also cured a merchant of Rajagir who was suffering from a disease of the head for seven years. He made him lie down on a couch, strapped him to it, cut open the skin of his head, opened a suture in the skull, drew out two living creatures and showed them to the people. He then closed the suture of the skull, stitched the skin of the head and applied some ointment. The man was cured in three weeks. (*ibid.*, pp. 386-88.)

2. *Manussattaṃ liṅgasampatti, hetu satthāradassanaṃ/ Pabbajjā guṇasampatti, adhikāro ca chandatā/ Aṭṭhadhammasamodhānā, abhinīhāro samijjhati// Bu.*

3. Parajika Atthakatha, Vol. II (V.R.I. edition) pp.40-41.

Eḷakassa ca nipannokāse tassa mātā vā pitā vā arahā vā paṇdukāsāvaṃ pārupitvā nipanno hoti. So rattibhāge āgantvā "Eḷakam māremī"ti mātaraṃ vā pitaraṃ vā arahataṃ vā māreti. "Imaṃ vatthuṃ māremī"ti cetanāya atthibhāvato ghātako ca hoti, anantariyakammaṃ ca phusati, pārājikaṃ ca āpajjati. Añño koci āgantuko nipanno hoti, "Eḷakaṃ māremī"ti taṃ māreti, ghātako ca hoti pārājikaṃ ca āpajjati, ānantariyaṃ na phusati. Yakkho vā peto va nipanno hoti"Eḷakaṃ māremī"ti taṃ mareti ghātakova hoti, na cānantariyaṃ phusati, na ca pārājikaṃ āpajjati, thullccayaṃ pana hoti. Añño koci nipanno natthi, eḷakova hoti, taṃ māreti, ghātako ca hoti, pācittiyaṃ ca āpajjati.'Mātāpituarahantānaṃ aññataraṃ māremī'ti tesaṃyeva aññataram māreti, ghātako ca hoti, ānantariyaṃ ca phusati, pārājikaṃ ca āpajjati. 'Tesaṃ aññataraṃ māressāmī'ti aññaṃ āgantukaṃ māreti, yakkhaṃ vā petaṃ vā māṛeti, eḷakaṃ vā māreti, pubbe vuttanayena veditabbaṃ. Idha pana cetanā dāruṇā hotīti

...Yo hi "lohitakaṃ asiṃ vā sattiṃ vā pucchissamī"ti palālapuñje pavesento tattha nipannaṃ mātaraṃ vā pitaraṃ vā arahantaṃ va āgantukapurisaṃ vā yakkhaṃ vā petaṃ vā tiracchānagataṃ vā māreti, vohāravasena "ghātako"ti vuccati, vadhkacetanāya pana abhāvato neva kammaṃ phusati, na āpattiṃ āpajjati.

4. *The Book of the Discipline,* p.281.
5. *Ibid.*, pp. 270-71.
6. *Ibid.*, p. 279.
7. *It-sing* (Travel Accounts).

Chapter 16

Bioethics and Indian Culture

Nirbhai Singh

1. Introduction

This chapter purports to focus attention on Bioethics and Indian culture, values and their relevance in the contemporary scenario. In the age of science and technology, search for global peace and justice seems to be a wild goose chase. Clouds of terrorism are hovering over our heads. Humanity is burning in the cauldron of violence and religious fanaticism and bigotry. The volcanic eruption of atomic bomb may usher in dooms day at any moment. Human beings may perish and God will have to restart the process of creation *de novo*. Oswald Spengler in his classical work *The Decline of The West* envisages that science and technology cannot yield any spiritual healing to the moral and spiritual needs of humanity.

From the very beginning, an important and never exhausted point of discussion has been the concept of *quality of life;* focusing on those problems which modern medicine could solve, in order to grant the highest health standards to the largest possible number of people. It, then, enjoins upon me to explain the concept of bio-ethics. This is a new branch of bioethics that has come up in the philosophical circles. It focuses on ethical aspect of human life for improving upon moral quality of life in society. It makes doctors of aware of their moral obligations. It takes up vital ethical and social issues. In fact, the new technologies give man such a power of intervention on man himself and environment never seen before; a power so huge that regulation and supervision are needed, both on research and utilization level. Van Rensselaer Potter, ecologist at the University of Wisconsin, in his book "*Bioethics*", coined the term "bioethics" in 1970. *A Bridge To The Future*", is based on a reflection on the risks of man's self-destruction due to unethical use of biotechnological inventions and discoveries. From then on, bioethical centres have multiplied the world over. New biomedical technologies have launched vigorous endeavour for better life and health.

Environmental ethics or Bioethics is an abortive attempt for healing the ailing humans. Both are illegitimate byproducts of modern technology and science. In the modern philosophical debates and seminars bioethics dominates. Science and technology have given birth to many incurable diseases. For example, cancer is incurable till today. It has distorted the Greek concept of *euthanasia* as mercy killing. In the original sense, it was used for heroic death. Modern medical science has taken a lame excuse for finishing the cancerous patient with an injection who may die peacefully. From ethical standpoint, it is immoral. Euthanasia was the key concept of the heroic societies. In the *Ramayana* and the *Mahabharata* heroic life was the anchor of *dharma* (righteous deed). The heroes of the epics are symbols *dharma*. Islam and Sikhism adopted it for expounding the concept of martyrdom, supreme sacrifice for the cause of truth. Similarly, many other cultural values of India have been destroyed. Aboriginal culture of the tribal people is crushed. Indigenous art of the tribal people is withering away due to technological waves.

In fact, the new technologies give such a power of intervention on man himself and environment, which was never seen before. It is based on a reflection on the risks of man's self-destruction due to a biotechnological delusion of omnipotence. Bioethical centres have multiplied throughout the world, taking up different positions but almost everywhere pointing out new hopes for a better future. We can thank new biomedical technologies along with risks.

In this era of post-modernity human destiny is in the melting volcanic pot of material values. Western materialistic outlook of science and technology has a satanic impact in all walks of life. In spite of these malignant influences, there are some redeeming rays of hope, which may help humanity in bridging the yawning gulf of survival and annihilation. No doubt, the Western civilization has imposed materialistic outlook on our lifestyle, but it could not dominate the essential Indian spiritual culture. I can concede this much that in our day-to-day interpersonal relations, we have evinced materialistic attitude towards the world and others but the collective psyche of the common folks of India is still tied up with its hoary spiritual culture.

Contemporary environmental ethics has focused on criticizing the anthropocentric and instrumental value theories of humanism, which develop around modern Western philosophy and upon securing non-anthropocentric viewpoints based upon the truth that both human beings and nature have equal values of life.

Indian philosophy and Confucianism have monistic viewpoint about the relationship between man and nature, existence and values, subject and object. It is an endeavour to overcome the dichotomy between fact and value, subject and object. Values do not endow to the object. Nothing is intrinsically added to the objective facts at all. Values are human creation. God is an anthropocentric value. He is incessantly transformed into non-anthropocentric formless Being (*nirankara*). Values also transcend anthropocentric aspect and culminate in non-anthropocentric monism.

Value creation carries out through self-cultivation. Thus, philosophy of self-cultivation is the meeting point of Indian philosophy and Confucianism. Monistic philosophy is the natural outcome of self-cultivation. In the Western philosophy reason is the main source of knowledge, while in Confucianism and Indian philosophy moral nature (*dharma*) serves as the source for the sublimation of life as the unification of human nature and existence. Reason posits a dichotomy of the subject and the object whereas self-cultivation dissolves it. In short, self-cultivation actualizes the value of *ren* (humanity) by overcoming the material desires. (*sannyasa*). Thus, Indian philosophy and Confucianism are inclusive humanism free from anthropocentricism.

2. Uniqueness of Indian Culture

What is spirituality? The uniqueness of Indian spirituality is that it gives scientific spiritual discipline of *yoga* (yoking to the Numinous), which is the basis of different schools of thought in Indian philosophy. The *Gita* is the key of Indian spiritual philosophy and culture, which is its practical dimension and the *Samkhya* system, is its theoretical base. Both put together constitute perfect voluntarist philosophy of life. Spiritual discipline (*sadhana*) concentrates on *rarefaction* of consciousness through different stages of *yoga*. It is transformation of the self from the empirical self to the eternal self without dissolving man's 'personal identity'. It is transformation from *natura naturata* to *natura naturans*. In other words, the *jiva* is transmuted into *atman*. The empirical gross self is transformed into the subtle self—'self-consciousness' (*viveka buddhi*). Thus, our concept of spirituality does not negate the empirical world; rather embraces it.

Spirituality does not have any ontic being like the Platonic ideas. It is a lived experience of consciousness. When consciousness is rarefied, it culminates in self-consciousness. In the mystic terminology of *Sufism*, it is ascent (*miraj*) of consciousness towards approximation to the supreme Reality. The highest state of transcendence is ecstasy. The mystic is at once in a state of eternity and temporality. In the medieval terminology of the saints and the *gurus* it is called *sahaj*.

It needs strenuous training and discipline for taming the mind. Indian culture emphasizes on cultivation of consciousness. Control of mind (*mana*) is the essence of Indian culture. *Sadhana* (spiritual discipline) is a means for it. Guru Nanak in one of his hymns in

"*The Japuji*" avers, "He who conquers his mind (consciousness), achieves victory over the worldly seductions". From Guru Nanak to Guru Gobind Singh 'martial culture' was developed. The Gurus exploited heroic and tribal spirit of the Indian heritage. It represents the spirit of the Indian culture. Material things are only means for creating heroic culture. It is cultivation of the self from within. Taming of the nature with material tools is civilization. In nutshell, freedom and culture are interchangeable terms.

A sharp contrast between Indian and Western standpoints is the subjectivist inward individual's autonomy as the supreme moral criterion *vis-à-vis* utilitarianism, contractualism, anarchism, and behaviourism. In this case, the Western fundamental reference is the concept of *person*, as the unique and irreproducible dualism of body and spirit. In the Indian culture, both body and spirit are reducible through self-cultivation to monism of the cosmic consciousness controlled by the cosmic law (*rita*). The study of human person, the meaning of life, and his specific nature is the basis of bioethics. Hence, the Western and Indian culture are poles apart.

Uniqueness of Indian culture lies in the fact that it does not advocate possessiveness of property and power. The Western culture is antipodes to it. It is science and technology oriented. Wealth or money is a part of power. It corrupts human mind. The menace of global terrorism is the necessary outcome of it. Use of power for selfish purposes is to be avoided. We are facing this crisis in day-to-day life. Indian culture advocates sense of disinterested attitude towards both wealth and power, and pleads for distanced involvement in the societal relations. This is meaning of *nishkama karma* of *the Gita* and *subha karma* of Guru Gobind Singh.

It is to be cultivated by de-schooling and re-schooling. The former process is emptying the mind of dead and morbid beliefs and concepts, which are acquired from the parents and other fellow beings. The latter is a process of indoctrinating new beliefs, ideas, ideologies, etc. The saints and the *gurus* played this significant role. Culture is cultivation of the self from within and taming of the nature with material tools is civilization.

Cultivation of mind is self-taming through education, which aims at freeing the self from the fetters of the worldly seductions. Freedom and culture are interchangeable terms. *Moksha* and *nirvana* connote emancipation of the self from attachment with the world. At the transcendental level, one enjoys eternal freedom. Paulo Freire talks of education and freedom in society. He ventilated his ideas in his works, *Cultural Action for Freedom* and *Pedagogy of the Oppressed*. These are *par excellence* works on education and culture. Decolonization opens gates for true liberation of methods of learning pedagogy— de-schooling and reschooling. Freire repeatedly emphasizes to imbibe the capacity for transcending what is merely given and purely determined.[2] Man's ultimate goal of action is to realize in praxis. Radical indoctrination of mind through education transforms or revolutionizes the existing social order. This is carried out through language, education and practical action.

The dominance of material values, in the age of science and technology, is the beginning of the annihilation of humanity. Matter has the potent quality of attraction whereas the spiritual values lay emphasis on ascent of the mind from the tentacles and seductions of the mundane world. Material values relegate spiritual values to the periphery. Hence, the present crisis of globalization technology *vis-á-vis* cultures and civilizations or of the East and the West has come to the fore. Science and industry have caused havoc and immense misery to humanity. They cannot yield peace and harmony in the world. Sufferings of human beings are increasing day and night. Humanity is being dragged towards annihilation. Indian spiritual values and culture are the only redeeming hopes of humanity.

The age of science and technology is the beginning of the end of humanity. Science and industry have caused immense misery to humanity. It is just a mirage (*mriga trishna*). From the point of view culture, there is nothing good or desirable about scientific knowledge. We are living on the hope that every cloud has a positive aspect. Need of the hour is revival of Indian cultural values in practical life. It is unfortunate that people are doggedly falling into trap of the scientists.

The material progression is delusive. The idea of great civilizational progress is a delusion, along with the hope that the truth will be known in the future. No doubt, science is good to a limited extent. Beyond certain limits, it is injurious for humanity. It has taught us how to fly in the skies, dive deep into the oceanic waters, but it has not taught us how to live peacefully on the earth along with other human beings.

In the light of the above given global gloomy and dismal picture of the world, it will be pertinent to discourse Indian culture and values (*dharma*) which survived through the ages. It is a historical fact that Egypt, Sumaria, Greece, Persia and other fountainheads of civilizations perished, but Indian civilization survived through the epoch of history. This credit goes to the spiritual values of Indian culture which are treasured in the traditions, ethos, the *Vedas*, *Puranas, Upanishads*, the *Gita*, Buddhist literature, the *epics* (The *Ramayana*, The *Mahabharata*, etc.), and in the medieval Bhakti literature). Then a question arises: what is the spirit of the culture? It is not concerned with the progression of civilization. It surrounds the civilization. The spirit of civilization lies in its unity and continuity.

It is true that wisdom of India is found in the scriptures and oral traditions, but we have wasted time in garnering chaff instead of grain. The scriptures are the *Vedas*, but we have wasted time binding the manuscripts. The central linchpin of the sacred scriptures is "life" which the scriptures, the epics and the traditions emphasize, but we have spent time in concealing the ciphers in them with exegetical expositions and explanations, which remain at superficial level.

3. What is Culture?

I am trying to explore philosophical dimensions of the Indian culture and values that emphasize its dynamic and heroic nature that mirrors the essence of Indian philosophy. Since time immemorial, Indian culture passed through vicissitudes of social progression and retrogression, but it retained its *sui generic* identity.

The medieval period was the decline of the Indian culture. India lost her cultural glory and spiritual values. Material and temporal values overshadowed its spiritual values. The Islamic culture overshadowed our culture and values in all walks of life.

The ancient and the medieval epochs are interlinked because culture and civilization are continuous processes and are the outcome of the primitive culture-forms to the civilized society. They need conceptual interlacing into a unity for having a holistic perspective on the Indian culture. The medieval India was dismal for want of religious fervour and human values. In the medieval India, religion played vital role in carrying forward past cultural heritage. Our culture was partially diminished owing to alien invasions. The medieval *Bhakti* movement condemned ritualism and formalism, which were devoid of real religious or prophetic spirit in theory and praxis. The medieval Bhaktas and the Sikh Gurus made supreme sacrifices and struggled hard to revive and retain the essence of ancient spiritual culture.

The aspirant has to develop inner urge to realize his real self. For this purpose, he needs a mentor to guide him. Spiritual mentor (*guru*) is the symbol of wisdom for mentoring him. The spiritual mentor encourages the traveller to undertake inner journey that leads him to self-discovery. Nevertheless, he himself has to take the journey. This is the central linchpin of the Indian culture

When the aspirant starts his pilgrimage, his vision gets wider and sharper; and gradually the limits of the phenomenal world vanish. Fear of death lurks in his inner mind withers away. His courage strangulates fear of death that paralyses mind. 'Leap of Faith' awakens him to the life of choice of freedom. He can discharge *nishkama karmas.*

The mentor's 'wise eyes' inspire to undertake life full of strife. Without suffering and obstacles, life is passivity, which does not motivate to reach out the 'Beyond', the real purpose of human life. Precondition of "beginner's mind on inner pilgrimage" is to still and empty our mind of all entices of the world and resolve all conflicts. Stilled mind in meditation awakens to vision of truth. Strong will-power overcomes failures. Failures kindle faith in truth.

Only genius and talented man visualises new emerging higher visions. This inward journey cannot be possible without emptying mind of the worldly attachments and strong will to achieve eternal truth. Fortification of will and knowledge are supplementary factors. Failures kindle faith in truth and strong will defeats failures. This is the spirit of dynamic view of Indian life.

Stilled and purified vision of truth of the mystics echoes *cosmic* music ("*anahad-nada*") of eternity. To realize it is fraught with many challenges and obstacles. For achieving this target, natural talent is to be coupled with acquired skill and strenuous steadfast striving (*sadhana*) for autonomous life. The sage realises it and thousand others can take clue from his life. We can sum up the argument: evergreen stream of life flows with spiralling states of consciousness surging to the eternity. Wisdom lies in flowing with the flowing stream of eternity that is attuned to the cosmic law from within and without.

Man is born imperfect in the world within the narrow walls of egocentric self (*jiva*). If the 'I' is to be true to my authentic and unique self, it needs to transcend the illusion of 'me'. He is to come out of it and identify himself with 'others' and the cosmic Self. In the beginning, he is oblivious of the oceanic consciousness. For voluntarist life, consciousness is to be dominated by will. This is the secret of heroic life and culture.

'Others' become 'I', yet also remain the 'not-I.' It implies distinct and independent nature of 'others'. When the 'I' remains as a distant observer, the 'I' sees only the manifest behaviour in the society. Nevertheless, when the 'I' identifies itself with its inner self, the 'I' becomes fully realized and perfect. From the mundane point of view, it is distancing oneself from others. The 'I' identifies myself with others' anxieties, greed, or their whole 'self'. I could not understand myself in forlornness, aloneness, alienation, hope or love.

For perfecting himself, the hero is to struggle in the world. He is to transform his imperfect self (*jiva*) into perfect self (*atman*). Self-transcendence from the limits of the empirical world and distanced involvement in it is the essence of Indian culture. It does not imply actual withdrawal from the worldly responsibilities, but inward detachment from it. One is to grapple with ordeals of the world with disinterested involvement and live life of continuous striving till the claws of death strangulates him.

The conceptual framework of the heroic culture and spiritual values is preserved in the repositories of the sacred *Vedic* and the Buddhist scriptures. The medieval devotional literature of the *bhaktas* and the *gurus* is replete with heroic culture and martial values. They created a new composite and heroic culture and values. Urge for transcending the fear of death is the natural offshoot of it. Transformation implies awakening the self to free will. When man plunges into adventurous life, it gives birth to heroic view of life and culture

Man is an animal and creative being, but he is distinct from the lower species. Culture tames and transforms the beast in him for making it a creative being. He is the only species, which can create the worldview with tools of language. For this purpose, he creates the worldview. He creates his own world of the values and strives to live according to them. He tries to translate these values in use. This is the purpose of human life. His basic objective is to have complete harmony with the Nature and other fellow beings.

My 'I' is to be attuned to the very essence of the real self. This is realization of the *'personal identity'* of man and his autonomy. Authentic self mirrors freedom that is the central linchpin of man in the world. The personal identity is not a given fact. It is to be cultivated with meditative continuous striving both from within and without. From within he advances to autonomy of the self and from without he socializes himself in the society. The inward journey of the self terminates when the 'I' realizes that I am a drop of water on the crest of the oceanic waves. I am concerned with others not as an observer, but as an active participant and co-traveller in the existential predicaments. They ushered in Cultural Revolution in India and prepared the nation to confront alien incursions. They identified themselves with the subaltern for their emancipation. They formulated egalitarian ideology for the welfare of the subaltern populace. This is existential and concrete view of man of the *medieval bhaktas* and the Sikh Gurus. The scholars have not highlighted this aspect.

Culture is the undercurrent of inner life of the collective psyche of the people. It is the secret that is preserved as 'ciphers' in the sacred scriptures. Being a lived experience, it can be realized by the intuitive mind. Mystic or the religious celebrity is competent to understand it. Philosophical analysis can crystallize the concepts, which are the undercurrents. From this standpoint, philosophical study of culture is justified. Since no comprehensive work has been done in this field, this chapter may inspire the researchers to go deep into the problem.

The western researchers have done work from their own perspectives. The philosophical understanding of the Indic culture from the Indian perspective is the central problem of this chapter. Culture, being a lived experience, is very difficult to understand for the 'outsiders'. It is difficult for them to penetrate into the citadel of others' onto-theology and ethos, and traditions. Similarly, the 'outsiders' cannot easily grasp the Indic scriptures and the cultural traditions. In addition, Indian scholars have not given a serious thought to the problem. Ceaseless endeavour is needed for presenting coherent and systematic philosophical picture of the culture. Being 'insiders' the Indian thinkers with profound conceptual understanding of the scriptures can do justice to understand them from our cultural perspective.

The Europeans were masters of the world during colonization period. For the last three hundred years, they dominated the world cultures. They introduced education loaded with Western culture and religious ideology. Education is always goal-oriented. There is no neutral education. It is either for domestication or for freedom of man (*cf.* Paulo Freire, *Cultural Action for Freedom,* p. 9). Education is the key to recuperation of the mystified reality. In the medieval period, Indian culture was "culture of silence" because Indians lacked freedom of expression. In the present research work, I propose to highlight the contribution of the medieval intellectual celebrities and the religious dignitaries who revived Indian culture. They had freedom of expression. They expressed their ideas without any fear. In the medieval period, we were not free to express our native culture.

In the field of conceptual framework of philosophy of culture, Indian scholars have been exegetically explaining it from the perspectives of linguistics (philology, semantics, etymology, semiotics, etc.), sociology, anthropology, sculpture, architecture, etc. These tools are useful for exposing and explaining literal meanings of the texts. From the philosophical standpoint, cultural understanding in the area of the proposed study is irrelevant. We have been explaining Indian culture with traditional linguistic tools. Western scholars, especially the German philologists, have done researches on the sacred scriptures. They claim that they are masters of Sanskrit and are competent to understand the Sanskrit texts. Their works are mostly concerned with preparing dictionaries, mythological indices, concordances, literal translations of the scriptures, etc. Their translations are done from the Christian standpoint. Their coloured explanations of the sacred texts have presented distorted picture of the Indian culture. They did not have in-depth understanding of the Indian ethos, traditions, conventions and customs. They provided improvised material. Philosophical perspective escaped their studies. Thus, our objective conceptual understanding of the Indian culture is lagging far behind. We are still living in the medieval ages. Our understanding of Indian culture is that of ropedancers. We have been interpreting Indian culture from the Western perspective. The lenses of Eurocentric methodology shadow our interpretations. It is unfortunate that Indian religious discourses continue limping along Hindu *Ashramas, Siddha* or *Yogi Mathas,* Sikh *Gurdwaras*, Muslim mosques, *Shivadwaras,* Jaina *Mandirs,* and *Buddhist Pagodas/ Stupas*.

Eurocentric methodology and hermeneutical contribution of the Jews to the Christian sacred scriptures is significant. Being 'outsiders', the Westerners cannot do full justice to our cultural heritage. The native Indians have been experiencing it since times immemorial. They breathe in cultural fragrance of the Indian soil day and night. Western interpretations of our texts are overshadowed with their conscious or unconscious cultural prejudices. It is very difficult to interpret culture of 'others' because they are alien. Nevertheless, there is no harm in using Eurocentric methodology. But it should be modified which should fit in with the indigenous culture of the land.

Since sixth century Christian era, influence of foreign languages (Arabic, Persian, English, etc.) cannot be denied. In addition to it, we have been aping the Westerners for the last three hundred years. The prevailing knowledge of the English knowing Indian elite is of the post-colonized impact. It is unfortunate that we have not come out of their domination though they have trivialized our culture, religion, and philosophy. They claim that they are experts to interpret Indian culture. We could not dispense with English language. It is said that language is the 'house of culture'. All ideas and concepts are preserved in the sacred repertoires. The Westerners have studied them from their limited perspectives. Max Muller, Monier-Monier Williams, Ernest Trumpp, B. Walker, H.H. Wilson and many others have presented lopsided and distorted picture of Indian thought and culture.

Precondition of interpreting others' culture is the sound grasp of Indian culture with critical and creative mind. One is to put aside one's prejudices and appreciate other's perspective. They are to abide by the objective rules of hermeneutics and logic. Lavish repeated quoting from the texts does not reveal creativity. Innovation of new ideas is the outcome of creative mind. The lenses of Eurocentric methodology have shadowed the interpretation of Indian culture. My endeavour is to interpret the Indian culture from the standpoint of Indian cultural milieu.

In earlier studies of Indian culture, emphasis was on historical and philological approaches/methods. Now there is a shift on the coeval Philosophical hermeneutics of social sciences and culture. In the modern times, emphasis is on interdisciplinary symbiotic method of studying culture, religion and other social disciplines. It includes historical, sociological, psychological, philological and exegetical tools and techniques. Nevertheless, history provides improvised data of persons, dates and places, but these are interpreted for working out philosophy of culture. Similarly, philological method takes us to the roots and semantics of the words. Many words travelled from Greece after Alexander's incursion in 320 BC. When the Arabs and the Persians came to India, after the seventh and the eighth centuries, many words travelled from Arabia and Persia. They changed their phones and meanings to adjust to the new cultural milieu of India. Their core meanings were wrapped in new languages. These will provide raw materials on which the world picture of our culture can be built.

It is hoped that our scholars will develop distinct tools for presenting Indian culture. They are to abide by objective rules of language. Lavish quoting from the texts does not show creativity. It requires creative and critical mind. I hope this study will stimulate the minds of the elite of India and abroad. If this shift sets in new trend of critical and analytical understanding of Indian culture and values it shall be at par with the Western cultural and civilizational advances. It will strengthen our faith, which anchors on sandy ground of irrational beliefs and traditions.

It may be pointed out here that the Indians did not have a sense of historical time. When the Arabs and the Turks came to India, the Indians developed sense of time. In Sikhism, Guru Nanak, the founder of Sikh faith showed practical sense of time, which other Gurus continued. Guru Gobind Singh's creation of the *Khalsa-panth* is the outcome of it.

It is difficult to tease out veridical information from scattered manuscripts that can be treated as benchmark for articulating the Indian culture. We are standing on a volatile point. If the materials available are philosophically interpreted, our perspective of Indian culture will be changed.

The material is scattered in different manuscripts, books, journals and traditions. The material on the ancient and the medieval periods pertaining to social, religious, political, and other areas is not available in compact form. It is because no critical and systematic research has been done. The materials are available in scanty form. Most of the works in the Muslim period available are written from the Qur'anic and the Semitic (Islamic) standpoints.

The Indian researchers are seemingly oblivious of the Semitic philosophical framework of the Semitic scriptures and the traditions.

No systematic relevant material is available on philosophical perspective. The works of Muslim scholars have Islamic bias and the Indian scholars suffer from their religious myopia. Their works are lopsided because they lack holistic perspective of the medieval era. If an Indian scholar writes, his perspective shall be either Vedantic or Buddhistic because both were dominating religious traditions of India. The Sikh scholar may be swayed in either the Vedic or the non-Vedic stream. If you want to present a holistic medieval world-view, a balanced and rational viewpoint will be an objective perspective. A comprehensive picture shall emerge if the Indic and the Semitic perspectives are taken together. From this point of view, the original works on the medieval religions, history, culture and philosophy are being perused for articulating coherent Indian culture and values. .

This chapter is dyed in the vision of secrets of dynamic view of life and the heroic Indian culture. It will inspire the readers for brooding and culling subtle meanings of the 'cipher' of Indian culture and the values that are life breath of our philosophical heritage scattered over the ages in the sacred literature and the religious and folk traditions. Indian culture inspires man for evincing strong will-power to come out of the muzzling conditions that were prevalent in the medieval India. One who has inherent 'strong desire' can go beyond to reach out his original source for regaining freedom and bliss.

The earlier researchers have not emphasized this aspect. The Sikh movement is the revival of 'cultural identity', which culminated in the creation of the *Khalsa*. The *Khalsa* ideology is representative of the militant social structure that reaffirms the heroic culture of India. Hence, one of the most significant contributions of the Gurus was to develop heroic culture of India. This is the philosophy of voluntarism, which the *Gita* propounded. The Gurus carried it forward. In the modern time, Mahatma Gandhi was the advocate of it.

Culture spirals round human life. Its nature and purpose is to mirror inner human life. Culture is a living and dynamic phenomenon that accompanies man from womb to tomb. It is not a sheer concept, but a lived experience of inmost forms that are potential and actualized. The former are hidden forms, which come to the surface. The creative celebrities cull the hidden culture-forms. The world cultures oscillate between the two aspects. Progress of human history is from potential to actualization of culture-forms through chequered historical epochs. Thus, culture is its inner possibilities. Man hopes that one day he shall be successful in knowing the 'Beyond'. It is continuous progression from chaos to unity, and from ignorance to knowledge. We are trying to transcend our *finitude* for becoming one with the Numinous. It is existential approach to culture. The temporal and the eternal are clubbed together in theory and practice.

Culture is a system of the pattern and modes of aspirations and expressions of values, institutionalization of life in society. It is an attitude and mode of dealing with objective reality and subjective personality. Three points are noteworthy in understanding perspectives on culture. First, culture is human creation. Second, it provides 'objective reality' and 'subjective interpretation' while churning the ideals, values, ideology, and so forth. Third, it represents interpersonal relationships for harmony and justice. It endeavours for adjustment that emanates from spontaneity and freedom of action. One can formulate new value system for bettering the existent social order. Here revival of Indian culture means restoration of freedom and self-dignity of man. This determines cultural identity of India.

If we go deep into the meaning of the term 'culture,' we will find that it is concerned with mind or consciousness. Culture is a principle of interlacing society into a unity. It brings connectivity between hearts and minds of the people in multi-cultured composite society of India. It is not primarily concerned with external progression of civilization. It is concerned with progression of the inner self (*atman*).

Now the philosophical questions arise: is culture divine

creation? What is the spirit of the culture? What is the concept of spirituality? Is Indian culture spiritual or non-spiritual? What is uniqueness of spiritual Indian Culture? What is the distinct cultural identity of India? Can it be motivated and learned? It means that *atman* (consciousness) is representative of Indian 'culture'. If we go into etymologies of the term 'culture' in Latin ('*cultura*') and German (*kultur*), (Arabic—*tahjib*), we find that both emphasize on cultivation of mind. Culture in Sanskrit language is *sanskriti*, which means cultivation of mind. It is said that "*atma ce sanskrite*" (consciousness is culture). The term *atma* stands for consciousness. Consciousness guides all human activities. At the initial stage, beastly desires dominate the sensuous self. These are refined by spiritual discipline

Culture (*sanskriti*) is cultivation of mind for fashioning its beastly, barbarian and uncivilized nature. It can be extended to society. Therefore, culture is a way of life of the people including their attitude towards other people and the world. Attitude implies values, beliefs, arts, aesthetic sense of sensibility, vision of social ideals, or values, etc. Cultural patterns of life are acquired in the society. These are mirrored through values, beliefs, and religious ways of living.

Suppression of culture does not mean annihilation of values, but the disappearance of certain means of expressing values. Expressions may change but the values once created become lasting. Once they are created in time, they transcend time. No culture dies. Thus, values are eternal and are for the ages to come. In this sense culture, which deals with network of values, is eternal and its spirit in the form of ideas and ideals hovers over heads of the people.

Culture is like an epic, which represents spirit of human life in a particular country. No one will be there to observe the progress of a "culture as an epic". Epic is a written prophecy. One can foresee one's death (ideology) in the future as an inevitable phenomenon, but no one is definite about its exact form. Thus, culture is to live in the blending of past, present and future into the 'eternal present'.

Man creates culture. It is not a divine creation. It is always in flux or 'becoming'. Spengler and Goethe are of the view that every culture passes through the epochs of history of the individual man. Ancient Vedic and the medieval periods are the blossoming phases of the Indian culture. Old cultures become a heap of rubbles and finally a heap of ashes, but spirit hovers over the ashes. History of cultures of the world reveals that cultures recycle in the progressive process of history. New cultures are rebuilt on the debris of old cultures.

The concept of progress may be linear or cyclic. It is primarily based on the cyclic view of time and the concept of time is a 'universal flux'. Disappearance of a culture does not imply annihilation of values, but temporary cessation of expression of means of expressing the values. The values are eternal but their expressions go on changing. The world cultural history oscillates between progress and retrogression, but it continues forever. It is a lived existential experience, which needs cultivation of mind. It is evinced spiritual discipline. Reason and insight both put together can discern continuity between eternity and temporality. It is only the mystic or the genius that lives in the 'eternal present' and discerns its continuity. The genius brings out spirit of culture-forms in new forms and puts them to use in history. This is how the human history retrogresses and progresses in different epochs. This is not a straight and linear prophetic path, but a zigzagged circuitous journey of the global cultures.

4. Heroic Nature of Indian Culture

Heracleitus (480 B.C.) avers, "War [conflict] is the father of all things". This strife is the stuff of dynamic life. If life is an eternal conflict of head and heart, then the central problem of human life is to wriggle out of the tension of suffering and pleasure. Then the self will be attuned to the eternal bliss of the spiritual self (soul/ *atma*). Perhaps, the Buddha was the first thinker who made earnest endeavour in this direction. He tried to overcome the phantom of death and the perennial strings of sufferings. He started his quest to find out permanent solution of the tragic sense of life, but ended his journey in *nirvana* that goes beyond the empirical world. It should recycle after climbing to the apex of self-transcendence. The realized person should be always active in society for eradication of suffering humanity. The *Bhaktas* and the *Gurus* created this heroic dimension of Indian culture.

In the transitional period from ancient to medieval epochs emphasis has been laid on cognition and will (*samkalpa*) was relegated to the subordinate position. Fortified will-power paralyzes fear of death. Courage muzzles fear of death. Acquiring of courage and transcending the fear of death is the strenuous inward pilgrimage to the 'Beyond'. The purposeful self-transcending process, continuously expanding vision, spirally ascends to Eternity. It paves way of new culture. Persistence and strong will lead to emancipation and autonomy of the self for discharging *nishkama karma* (categorical imperative). This chapter lays emphasis on heroic aspect of culture, which has roots in the tribal primitive traditions of the land. Heroic values are the necessary outcome of the heroic culture. It anchors on dynamic view of life, which advocates continuous striving for perfecting man in the world and discharging his worldly responsibilities.

An endeavour will be made to portray development of our culture through the vicissitudes of ancient and medieval epochs. In the medieval ages, Indian culture digressed to life-and-world-negation, dismal and pessimistic view of life. The medieval *Bhaktas* reaffirmed the status of the world and restored the *historical action* (*karma*). During medieval period, the *Bhaktas* and the *Gurus* developed historical sense of time. It added new dimension to the Indian culture. It rejuvenated voluntarism in Indian tradition. The heroic culture revisited with greater vigour and revolt. The *Bhaktas* bitterly castigated the existent social order that marginalized the subaltern folk. They steeled will of the subaltern marginalized populace so that they could confront boldly tyranny and rebel against inhuman atrocities. It was a movement of voluntarist culture. There was a powerful resurgence in cultural revival in India. The medieval *Bhaktas* emerged as a powerful counterforce. Thus, odysseys of the central theme will represent microscopic philosophical analysis of the concept of the Indian culture along with multidimensional aspects of social affirmation and restoration of historicity of human action that led to healthy ideology.

"To do, think and aspire is to be". The sage embraces the primordial one and becomes model for others. The Buddha rightly said "*atma dipo bhava*". It means that thousand candles can be lit from a single candle. This is the altruistic ideal of the world's living religions and cultures.

Our ancient sages refined the barbaric culture. The purpose of human life is to control the body for the sake of higher values which man creates for living a life of bliss (*anand*). When man controls his bodily person and lives life of human values, he is living real human life. Thus, the Sikh movement emphasizes on active resistance to evil and struggle in life. It fortified will of the Indians. It leads to heroic life in the world. The Gurus steeled will of the humiliated masses. They prepared martial heroes who were everready to stake their lives for the supreme sacrifice for the sake of higher values. They developed steadfast faith in the *Akalpurakh*.

Indian culture has its roots in the *Vedic* lore and the Shramanic indigenous traditions of Buddhism and Jainism. The *Vedic* and the Shramanic cultures intermingled on the Indian soil. Both represent dynamic cultures and dynamic views of life. They emphasize on quest for secrets and purposes of life and transcendence over death. It is a search for self-discovery and identification with 'others'. Inward journey takes one to the heart, which rebounds with prompting right path to truth (new realms). One is to live life of continuous striving for achieving new spirally ascending states of consciousness that flow with the ever-flowing stream of eternity. One is to make one's own efforts and the mentor is only to guide. With strong will-power, the aspirant develops 'intentional life' of autonomy and courage. It signifies voluntarism of Indian culture. It is a perennial universal problem of life. The 'others' are as real as 'I' am. They are 'persons' having autonomy of will.

REFERENCES

1. Member Indian Council Philosophical Research (ICPR), HRD Ministry, New Delhi.
   Res. Address : # Kothi-No.306/Lane-7, Jujhar Nagar, Patiala-147003/ Phon.0175-2372956: Mob. 9463940721 : email addresses; nbspta@gmail.com, nbspta@yahoo.com.
2. *Cf.* Paulo Freire, *Cultural Action for Freedom,* Australia: Penguin Books, 1974, p. 9.

Chapter 17

Intellectual Property Rights : A Bird's Eye View

Rakesh Kumar Sinha

Intellectual property refers to creations of the mind: inventions, literary and artistic works, and symbols, names, images, and designs used in commerce.

Intellectual property is divided into two categories: Industrial property, which includes inventions (patents), trademarks, industrial designs, and geographic indications of source; layout designs of integrated circuits and copyright, which includes literary and artistic works such as novels, poems and plays, films, musical works, artistic works such as drawings, paintings, photographs and sculptures, and architectural designs.

1. Industrial Property

1.1 Patents

The word 'Patent' comes from the latin '*litterae patentes*', meaning an open letter. The first recorded patent of invention was granted to John of Utynam. In 1449, he was awarded a 20-year monopoly for a glass making process previously unknown in England. In return, John was required to teach his process to native Englishmen.

That same function of passing on information is now fulfilled by the publication of a "patents specification."

Today a patent is an exclusive right awarded to an inventor to prevent others from making, selling, distributing, importing or using their invention, without licence or authorisation, for a fixed period of time (TRIPS stipulates 20 years minimum from filing date). In return, society requires that the patent applicant disclose the invention in a manner that enables others to put it into practice. This increases the body of knowledge available for further research. As well as sufficient disclosure of the invention, there are three requirements (although details differ from country to country) that determine the patentability of an invention: novelty (new characteristics which are not "prior art"), non-obviousness (an inventive step not obvious to one skilled in the field), and utility (as used in the US) or industrial applicability (as used in the UK).

1.2 Industrial Designs

Industrial designs protect the aesthetic aspects (shape, texture,pattern, colour) of an object, rather than the technical features. TRIPS requires that an original design be eligible for protection from unauthorised use by others for a minimum of 10 years.

1.3 Trademarks

Trademarks provide exclusive rights to use distinctive signs, such as symbols, colours, letters, shapes or names to identify the producer of a product, and protect its associated reputation. In order to be eligible for protection a mark must be distinctive of the proprietor so as to identify the proprietor's goods or services. The main purpose of a trademark is to prevent customers from being misled or deceived. The period of protection varies, but a trademark can be renewed indefinitely. In addition many countries provide protection against unfair competition, sometimes by way of preventing misrepresentations as to trade origin regardless of registration of the trademark.

1.4 Geographical Indications

Geographical Indications (GIs) identify the specific geographical origin of a product, and the associated qualities, reputation or other characteristics. They usually consist of the name of the place of origin. For example, food products sometimes have qualities that derive from their place of production and local environmental factors. The geographical indication prevents unauthorized parties from using a protected GI for products not from that region or from misleading the public as to the true origin of the product.

1.5 Trade Secrets

Trade secrets consist of commercially valuable information about production methods, business plans, clientele, etc. They are protected as long as they remain secret by laws which prevent acquisition by commercially unfair means and unauthorised disclosure.

2. Artistic and Literary Property

2.1 Copyright

Copyright grants exclusive rights to the creators of original literary, scientific and artistic works. Copyright only prevents copying, not independent derivation. Copyright protection begins, without formalities, with the creation of the work, and lasts (as a general rule) for the life of the creator plus 50 years (70 years in the US and EU). It prevents unauthorised reproduction, public performance, recording, broadcasting, translation, or adaptation, and allows the collection of royalties for authorised use. Computer programms are protected by copyrights, as software source and code have been defined as a literary expression.

2.2 Sui Generis Systems

2.2.1 Integrated Computer Circuits

A specific *sui generis* form of protection for the design of integrated computer circuits. As the inventive step is often minimal and originality is the only requirement, the minimum period of protection under TRIPS is 10 years.

2.2.2 Plant Breeders' Rights

Plant breeders' rights (PBRs) are granted to breeders of new, distinct, uniform and stable plant varieties. They normally offer protection for at least fifteen years (counted from granting). Most countries have exceptions for farmers to save and replant seeds, and for the use of protected materials for further breeding.

2.2.3 Database Protection

The EU has adopted legislation to provide *sui generis* protection in respect of databases, preventing unauthorised use of data compilations, even if non-original. Exclusive rights to extract or utilize all or a substantial part of the contents of the protected database are granted.

3. Indian Perspective

The importance of intellectual property in India is well established at all levels—statutory, administrative and judicial. India ratified the agreement establishing the World Trade Organisation (WTO). This Agreement, *interalia*, contains an Agreement on Trade Related Aspects of Intellectual Property Rights (TRIPS) which came into force from 1st January, 1995. It lays down minimum standards for protection and enforcement of intellectual property rights in member-countries which are required to promote effective and adequate protection of intellectual property rights with a view to reducing distortions and impediments to international trade. The obligations under the TRIPS Agreement relate to provision of minimum standard of protection within the member-countries legal systems and practices.

3.1 Legislative Initiatives

India is a signatory to the WTO Agreement and is required to align its laws on intellectual property rights in accordance with the obligations under the TRIPS Agreement of the WTO Agreement. Legislations conforming to obligations under the TRIPS Agreement, relating to 'Patents, Trademarks. Geographical Indications and Industrial Designs have been amended/enacted. As on date, these legislations are fully in compliance with its TRIPS obligations.

While amending/enacting these legislations, the opportunity was also utilized to modernize and revamp the legislations, incorporate provisions for simplification of procedures and protection of national/public interest. The Agreement provides for norms and standards in respect of all the forms of intellectual property.

3.2 Copyrights

India's copyright law, laid down in the Indian Copyright Act 1957 as amended by Copyright (Amendment) Act 1999, fully reflects the Berne Convention on Copyrights, to which India is a party. Additionally, India is party to the Geneva Convention for the Protection of rights of Producers of Phonograms and to the Universal Copyright Convention. India is also an active member of the World Intellectual Property Organisation (WIPO), Geneva and UNESCO. The copyright law has been amended periodically to keep pace with changing requirements. The recent amendment to the copyright law, which came into force in May 1995, has ushered in comprehensive changes and brought the copyright law in line with the developments in satellite broadcasting, computer software and digital technology. The amended law has made provisions for the first time, to protect performer's rights as envisaged in the Rome Convention Several measures have been adopted to strengthen and streamline the enforcement of copyrights. These include the setting up of a Copyright Enforcement Advisory Council, training programs for enforcement officers and setting up special policy cells to deal with cases relating to infringement of copyrights.

3.3 Trade Marks

Trade marks have been defined as any sign, or any combination of signs capable of distinguishing the goods or services of one undertaking from those of other undertakings. Such distinguishing marks constitute protectable subject matter under the provisions of the TRIPS Agreement. The Agreement provides that initial registration and each renewal of registration shall be for a term of not less than 7 years and the registration shall be renewable indefinitely. Compulsory licensing of trade marks is not permitted. Keeping in view the changes in trade and commercial practices, globalisation of trade, need for simplification and harmonisation of trade marks registration systems, etc., a comprehensive review of the Trade and Merchandise Marks Act 1958 was made and a Bill to repeal and replace the 1958 Act has since been passed by Parliament and notified in the Gazette on 30.12.1999. This Act not only makes Trade Marks Law, TRIPS compatibility but also harmonises it with international systems and practices. The subordinate legislation of the laws on Trade Marks have been modified.

3.4 Geographical Indications

The Agreement contains a general obligation that parties shall provide the legal means for interested parties to prevent the use of any means in the designation or presentation of a good that indicates or suggests that the good in question originates in a geographical area other than the true place of origin in a manner which misleads the public as to the geographical origin of the good. There is no obligation under the Agreement to protect geographical indications which are not protected in their country or origin or which have fallen into disuse in that country. A new law for the protection of geographical indications, viz., the Geographical Indications of Goods (Registration and the Protection) Act 1999 has also been passed by the Parliament and notified on 30.12.1999. The subordinate legislation of the laws on Geographical Indications has been modified.

3.5 Industrial Designs

Obligations envisaged in respect of industrial designs are that independently created designs that are new or original shall be protected. Individual governments have been given the option to exclude from protection, designs dictated by technical or functional considerations, as against acsthetic consideration which constitutes the coverage of industrial designs. The right accruing to the right holder is the right to prevent third parties not having his consent from making, selling or importing articles being or embodying a design, which is a copy or substantially a copy of the protected design when such acts are undertaken for commercial purposes. The duration of protection is to be not less than 10 years. A new designs law repealing and replacing the Designs Act 1911 has been passed by Parliament in the Budget Session 2000. This Act has been brought into force from 11.5.2001.

3.6 Patents

The basic obligation in the area of patents is that, invention in all branches of technology whether products or processes shall be patentable if they meet the three tests of being new, involving an inventive step and being capable of industrial application. In addition to the general security exemption which applied to the entire TRIPS Agreement, specific exclusions are permissible from the scope of patentability of inventions, the prevention of commercial exploitation of which is necessary to protect public order or morality, human, animal, plant life or health or to avoid serious prejudice to the environment. Further, members may also exclude from patentability of diagnostic, therapeutic and surgical methods of the treatment of human and animals and plants and animal other than micro-organisms and essentially biological processes for the production of plants and animals. The TRIPS Agreement provides for a minimum term of protection of 20 years counted from the date of filing. India had already implemented its obligations under Articles 70.8 and 70.9 of TRIP Agreement. A comprehensive review of the Patents Act 1970 was also made and a bill to amend the Patents Act 1970 was passed by Parliament on 14 May, 2002. The amendment to the Patent Law has been made operational from 20th May, 2003.

4. CSIR's Perspective

Since its inception in 1942, CSIR is dealing with Patents. But stimulating point was Haldi in 1995. Two US based Indians, S.K. Das and H.P. Cohly, were granted a US patent 1995 on "Use of turmeric in wound healing". This patent claimed the administration of an effective amount of turmeric through local and oral route to enhance the wound healing process, as a novel finding. CSIR has challenged this patent on the basis that this does not satisfy novelty criterion for the fact that this process is well known in India since ages. After lot of ups and downs, CSIR won the battle in 1997. It was first time that a patent based on the traditional knowledge of a developing country was challenged successfully and US Patent Office (USPTO) revoked the patent. CSIR thus learns and sets an international trend to challenge patents based on traditional knowledge. Encouraged by this, CSIR has fought the battle of Basmati in 1999 and won.

The onset of CSIR initiatives in IP domain was the articulation of IP policy in 1996. CSIR has adopted IP policy as "To maximize the benefits to CSIR from its intellectual capital by stimulating high level of innovation through a judicious system of rewards, ensuring timely and effective legal protection for its IP and leveraging and forcing strategic alliances for enhancing the value of IP and from its IP". CSIR has got reward of implementation of IP policy as it became first patent filer in India and eighth in PCT filing in world among publicly funded R&D organization. It has a patent portfolio of 1250 Indian patents and 1770 foreign patents.

In view of the fact that patent can be granted to anyone of any age, CSIR has given the slogan "catch them young". CSIR has launched an inventtion competition amongst Indian school children. The strategy of targeting the school kids was deliberately taken, as it had the indirect objective of creating an interest and awareness in IP amongst the teachers and parents as well.

5. Acknowledgement

The author is thankful to DG, CSIR for mentoring and inspiration.

[Dr. Rakesh Kumar Sinha has obtained Ph.D. in Ceramic Engineering in 1993 from Institute of Technology, Banaras Hindu University. He has nine years of research experience in advanced ceramic materials, seven years of industrial experience and for the last five years he is Scientist in Council of Scientific & Industrial Research (Ministry of Science & Technology), New Delhi. Presently he is attached with Director General, CSIR and Secretary to Government of India, Department of Scientific and Industrial Research. He underwent training on IPR in Japan. In addition he has completed DL 01 Certificate in Intellectual Property Rights from World Intellectual Property Organization (WIPO) also. He can be reached at rksinha@csir.res.in or rks_taurean@yahoo.com.]

Chapter 18

Intellectual Property

Sumit Siddharth

A scientist spending a major part of his/her life in a laboratory in search of something which is of mass benefit must be provided with certain rights or protections for his/her essential research. These rights, protections will be discussed in this chapter.

WIPO stands for World Intellectual Property Organization. It was established in 1967 as a specialized agency of United Nations with the sole motive of promoting the protection of intellectual property throughout the world. It needed different countries and many intellectual organizations to work together for the fulfilment of the above mentioned initiative.

A very interesting term "Intellectual Property" arises in the lines mentioned above. Before dealing with intellectual, it is necessary to lay emphasis on intellect. Literally speaking intellect means — the power to perceive, interpret, know and understand (*Webster's Student Dictionary of English Language*, International Encyclopedic edition Reprint 2006) the power of the mind to think in a logical manner and aquire knowledge (*Oxford Advanced Learner's Dictionary*, 5th edition Editor Crowther J., Oxford University Press).

Intellectual is a person of trained intelligence and knowledge or those whose work requires exercise of the intellect (*Webster's Student Dictionary of English Language*, International Encyclopedic edition, Reprint 2006). Intellectual is of or connected with a person's powers of reasoning (*Oxford Student Dictionary*, 5th edition, Editor Crowther J., Oxford University Press).

Property means any object that a person may lawfully acquire and own, any possession especially land or real state. (*Webster's Student Dictionary of English Language*, International Encyclopedic edition, Reprint 2006)

Consigning both these terms we find that Intellectual Property is a *subject of personal property which also includes trademarks, copyrights and trade secrets* (Intellectual Property by Jennifer Gordon). *Intellectual Property relates to Industrial property includes inventions, trademarks, industrial design and geographic indications of source whereas copyrights emphasises on literary and artistic works such as novels, poems and plays, films, musical works, drawings, paintings, photographs, sculptures and architectural designs.*

Intellectual property is the legal characterisation of biotechnological process example transformed microorganisms, developed improved varieties, etc. Intellectual Property Protection (IPP) and Intellectual Property Rights (IPR) are available to protect this property.

Intellectual Property is an abstract property against tangible (real) physical property which one can feel, see and use in physical forms.

License is the written or printed certificate of legal permit, it is a legal permit to do something (*Webster's Student Dictionary of English Language*, International Encyclopedic edition, Reprint 2006)

Licensed Intellectual Property includes patents, trademarks, trade-secrets, copyrights. All these terms will be dealt with but emphasis will be given to patents only.

Patent is a government protection to an inventor, securing to him for a specific time exclusive rights to his invention (*Webster's*

Student Dictionary of English Language, International Encyclopedic edition, Reprint 2006)

Patent is an official document giving the holder the sole right to make use, or sell an invention and preventing others from copying it (*Oxford Advanced Learner's Dictionary*, 5th edition, Editor Crowther J., Oxford University Press).

Patent is an exclusive right bestowed to the owner or possessor of an invention to make use, manufacture and market the invention providing the invention fulfils certain essential conditions mentioned in the law. In accordance with law patent is a proprietary right and, therefore, it can be sold, licensed, inherited, given away and also can be abandoned. In a more sophisticated way patents defend plans and schemes that provide functional explanation to certain uncertainty problem.

A patentee is a person enjoying a patent. The invention must be disclosed in a patent document by the patentee so that anyone can practice it after the expiration of the patent or practice it with the consent of the patentee during the life of the patent.

The law protecting patents in India is governed by "The Patent Act 1970." A patentable invention is a new and useful art, process, method or manner of manufacture, machine, apparatus or other article, or substance produced by manufacture and includes any new and useful improvement of any of them, and an alleged invention.

According to Indian Patent Act, an invention means a new product or process involving an inventive step and capable of industrial application. An invention must satisfy the following essential requirements for being patented.

Novelty

Global state of art constitute information appearing in magazines, technical journals, books, newspaper, etc. An invention is not considered novel if it forms a part of global state of art. An invention will not be novel if it has been disclosed in public through any type of publications anywhere in the world before filing a patent application for the invention. Prior use of invention and oral description of the invention in a conference or seminar before filing an application for patent can also destroy its novelty.

Non Obviousness

The differences between the prior art and the invention as a whole must have been unobvious to a person of ordinary skill in the art at the time the invention was made (*Intellfctual Property* by Jennifer Gordon). There must be an inventive step involved in the patent application. Inventive step means that the invention must not only be new but must also result from a creative idea which is non obvious. The complexity and simplicity does not have any effect on the grant of the patent.

Usefulness/Utility

For a patent to be granted, the invention must possess an element of utility in it. No valid patent can be granted for an invention devoid of utility. However the criterion of utility has recently been somewhat controversial in biotechnology related inventions.

Sufficiency of Disclosure

This requirement explains that the invention must be disclosed in sufficient detail so that the public can practice the invention once the patent has expired. Sufficiency of disclosure ensures that the public is benefited from the invention.

Patent Documents

There are two types of Patent Documents :

(i) *Provisional Specification :* A provisional specification need not contain full and specific description of the invention. A general description of the invention, its field of application and the anticipated results are sufficient for filing a provisional specification. When the invention is only at a conceptual shape and there will be occurring a delay in submitting full and specific description of the invention then the provisional specification is filed in. Provisional specification must be followed by complete specification for obtaining a patent for the invention.

(ii) *Complete Specification :* It is necessary to submit a complete specification for obtaining a patent. Complete specification must contain the title of the invention, field to which the invention belongs, full description of the invention, drawings if necessary, its operation, methodology of performing and claims explaining the scope of the invention.

In India, the term of the patent is 20 years from the date of filing for all types of inventions. The maintenance fee must be paid for maintaining the fee, if the maintenance fee is not paid, the patent will cease to remain in force and the invention becomes open to public.

Infringement of a Patent

Infringement is the act of violation or encroachment.

Someone using the subjecting matter claimed in a patent without the owner's approval or in disagreement with the terms of use given by the owner during the life of the patent infringes the patent. A person who make, uses or sells the patented invention is a direct infringer. Anyone actively encouraging others to make use or sell the patented invention without the consent of the owner is an indirect infringer. Anyone knowingly selling or supplying an item for which the only use is in connection with the patented invention is a contributory infringer.

- There occurs no infringement if the properties contained in the new product are altered and the new product can be patented freshly.
- Only the new properties of the new product can be patented and not the older ones.
- No infringement occurs during repairing of patented for the purpose of repair only. But making a new product for machine by interpretation during repair may be infringement.
- Any unauthorised selling of the patented apparatus, device, machine, part of whole substance can be under the act of infringement.

Copyright

Copyrights protect expressed materials, i.e., materials in printed, video recorded or in taped forms. Copyright protections is only a form of expression of ideas. In India, Copyright Act was amended in 1994 and brought enforce in 1999. It includes computer program, tables and databases. Copyrights in the area of Biotechnology includes databases of DNA and protein.

Tradesecrets (Knowhow)

The Private Proprietary Information that benefits the owners is called Tradesecrets (Biotechnology by R.C. Dubey). In the area of Biotechnology tradesecrets include hybridisation conditions, cell lines, processing, designing, etc.

Trademarks

Trademarks are the identification symbol used to distinguish the trader's goods from similar goods of other traders. For example IBM for computers, KODAK for photography goods.

Advantages of Patents and other forms of IPR are :

1. Patents and other IPR encourages the intellectual and artistic creations.
2. Patents and other IPR safeguards these intellectual and artistic creations.
3. Patents and other Intellectual Property Rights help in believing and spreading new ideas and technologies quickly and widely.
4. Patents and other IPR provide consumers with the result of creation and invention.
5. Provides increased opportunities for the distribution of the above effects across the countries in a manner proportionate to national levels of economic and industrial development. (OEDC, Paris, 1989)

Disadvantages of Patents

1. Things remained uncovered by patent can be misused.
2. Claims to be defended can be expensive.
3. Sufficient disclosure can be valuable to the competitors.

Dr. Ananda Mohan Chakrabarty (an Indian born American Scientist) created a Superbug using Pseudomonas putida strains which eats upon oil spices. But the superbug created by Ananda Mohan Chakrabarty was not patented because the US laws before 1980 did not allow the patent to living organisms. micro-organisms.

It was the year 1988 in United States of America when a patent was granted to "oncomouse", a genetically engineered mouse containing human cancer gene which was a living organism. Dr. Ananda Mohan Chakrabarty filed a case in US Supreme Court in 1990 and won it following which the US Government allowed him to treat oil spills by using Pseudomonas based superbug.

The below mentioned Biological Inventions can be patented :

1. Genetically modified organisms.
2. New organisms isolated.
3. Secondary metabolites.
4. Proteins and Enzymes.
5. Composition of the product.
6. The process of exploitation of micro-organisms to produce antibiotics.
7. Methods employed for obtaining industrial products.

NOTES

Gordon, J., "*Intellectual Property*."

Dubey, R.C., "*Biotechnology*".

OXFORD ADVANCED Learner's Dictionary, 5th Edition, Oxford University Press.

Patent Information Centre, Punjab State Council for Science and Tech , Chandigarh.

WEBSTER's Student Dictionary of English Language, International Encyclopedic Edition, Reprint 2006.

Chapter 19

Euthanasia : A Brief Survey

Madhubala Kumari

Euthanasia is a compound of two Greek words—'eu' and '*thanatos*'—meaning literally a 'good death'. Today 'Euthanasia' is generally understood to mean the bringing about of a good death 'mercy killing', where one person, *A* ends the life of another person *B*, for the sake of *B*. This understanding of Euthanasia emphasizes two important features of acts of Euthanasia :

1. It involves the deliberate taking of a person's life;
2. that life is taken for the sake of the person whose life it is—typically because he or she is suffering from an incurable or terminal disease.

This distinguishes euthanasia from most other forms of killing.

So, Euthanasia may be defined as an action in which a person is intentionally killed or allowed to die because it is believed that the individual would be better off dead than alive—or else, as in the case of irreversible coma, at least no worse off. Hence, in modern usage euthanasia has come to mean painless bringing about the death of a person who is suffering from a terminal or incurable disease or condition. Euthanasia, it is often argued, involves the deliberate or intentional termination of life. Administering a lethal injection, or withholding ordinary life sustaining means, are cases of intentional termination of life, withholding extraordinary means and allowing the patient to die.

Thus we can say that Euthanasia or mercy killing which was used as 'good death' in the Greek has come to be applied specifically in the medical field to the intentional killing of a human being for the purpose of ending his suffering or of removing some burden. However, it should be construed broadly so as to cover circumstances such as an accident, where an injured person asks a passerby to end his suffering by killing him, or a wounded soldier asks his commander to be 'put out of his misery'. The central moral considerations are the same whether or not the setting is professional or institutional, though the medical does raise specific questions of its own, such as what the role of a doctor should be? While the purpose of euthanasia, namely the ending of suffering or removal of a burden, is the one explicitly stated by most organizations that support legalization of the practice, we will see that other objectives are also evolved, and that these too need to be evaluated in the light of the philosophical ideas used to justify them.

Kinds of Euthanasia

Euthanasia can be classified as voluntary and involuntary, and as active and passive :

1. *Voluntary Euthanasia* : A competent, rational person requests or gives informed consent about a particular action or withholding of treatment that will lead to his or her death.
2. *Involuntary Euthanasia* : Bringing about people's death without their consent, although the consent of relatives may be obtained.
3. *Active Euthanasia* : Taking direct action, such as a lethal injection, to kill a person; also known as 'mercy killing'.

4. *Passive Euthanasia* : Allowing patients to die by withholding life support or medical treatment that would prolong their lives.

History of Euthanasia

Euthanasia in various forms is not a new practice in civilization. In ancient Sparta, those regarded as physically unfit for some purpose, or as incurably ill, or as useless to the state, were killed or allowed to die. In ancient Greece and Rome, the evidence suggests that deformed babies were 'exposed' or left to die. Such practice reached its heights hitherto unthinkable in Nazi Germany and in various Communist countries. It has most probably always been present in one or another part of the world.

But the fact that a social practice is common or even prevalent throughout the world, does not make it morally legitimate. Indeed, the revelation of the atrocities that took place as part of Hitler's 'euthanasia programme caused many nations of the world, particularly in the West, to recoil from the thought that it may be permissible for anyone, especially doctors or health-care workers, to kill or assist in the killing of an innocent person either because it was thought to be in that person's interests or in the interests of any one else, including society as a whole. It raises a great debate in favour and against the practice of Euthanasia.

Arguments given against the Practice of Euthanasia

There are many religions, philosophers and even branches of philosophy which are deadly against the practice of euthanasia in any form and they give their own reasons for that such as :

1. Aristotle believed that wilful euthanasia was very wrong. Virtue, he argued, requires that we face death bravely rather than take the cowardly way out by quitting life in the face of pain and suffering.

2. The Pythagoreans, who wrote the Hippocratic oath, also opposed euthanasia on the ground that the gods are our keepers and we are the possessions of the gods. To kill ourselves is to sin against the gods. As property of God, no human has the right to destroy his or her life or wantonly take the life of another. This understanding of human life as inherently precious and belonging to God has been immensely influential in the Jewish, Christian and Islamic views on euthanasia.
3. In the Jewish tradition, death should never be hastened; physicians who kill patients, even if their intention is to relieve pain and suffering are considered murderers.
4. According to Islamic religion, illness and suffering are part of God's will. Taking life interferes with God's will.
5. In Buddhist philosophy self-willed death, even in cases of suffering and pain, violates the principle of sanctity of life. It is also because ;
    - suffering is a means to work out bad *karma* rather than transferring it to the next life, and
    - a person who assists in suicide or performs euthanasia will be negatively affected by that participation.
6. Hinduism also teaches that suffering should be endured, because it allows us to work out negative *karma*. Those who deliberately shorten their lives will carry their negative *karma* into a later life.
7. The Dalai Lama teaches that: "Your suffering is due to your own *karma*, and you have to bear the fruit of that *karma* anyway in this life or another. Unless you can find some way of purifying it. In that case it is considered to be better to experience the *karma* in this life of a human where you have more abilities to bear it in a better way, than for example, an animal, who is helpless and can suffer even more because of that".
8. Most historians of Western morals argue that Judaism, and

the rise of Christianity contributed greatly to the general feeling that human life has sanctity and must not deliberately be taken. To take an innocent human life is, in these traditions, to usurp the right of God to give and take life. It has also been seen by influential Christian writers as a violation of natural law.

9. Even the great eighteenth century German philosopher Immanuel Kant who is of the opinion that moral truths are founded on reason rather than religion, nonetheless thought that "man cannot have the power to dispose of his life".

Thus we see these are the arguments given in favour of prohibition of euthanasia.

Arguments given in favour of the Practice of Euthanasia

In subsequent centuries, British philosophers notably David Hume, J. Bentham and J. S. Mill challenged the religious basis of morality and the absolute prohibition of suicide, euthanasia and infanticide. There are certain plausible arguments given in the defense of Euthanasia especially for assisted suicide and voluntary active euthanasia; they are as follows :

1. The contemporary debate on euthanasia has been influenced primarily by ancient Greek and Judeo-Christian views on death. Greek physician regarded health as a human ideal par excellence. Because human worth and social usefulness depended on one's state of health, chronically sick people were expendable. Their lives could be terminated with or without their consent.
2. Plato favoured euthanasia of deformed and sickly infants because they would be a burden on the polis.
3. The Roman philosopher Seneca and the early Stoics taught that human ought to quit life nobly when they are no longer socially useful.

4. If a person is suffering considerably pain due to an incurable illness, then that person's continued existence may very well not be in his or her own interest.
5. A person killing himself or herself in such circumstances may very well satisfy the following conditions :
   - It neither violates anyone else's rights, nor wrongs anyone; and
   - It does not make the world a worse place.
6. An action that satisfies (a) and (b) condition is not contrary to one's own interest, cannot be morally wrong.
7. Therefore, a person's committing suicide in such circumstances would not be morally wrong.
8. It could be morally wrong to assist a person to commit suicide only if either it was morally wrong for that person to commit suicide, or if commiting suicide in the circumstances described above.
9. Therefore, it would not be wrong to assist a person in the circumstances described above.
10. Whenever assisting a person in committing suicide is justified, voluntary euthanasia is also justified.
11. Therefore, voluntary active euthanasia would not be morally wrong in the circumstances described above.

Should Euthanasia be legalized?

Now here question arises if euthanasia is morally and ethically permissible, then should it be legalized? This question deserves more careful considerations; because even a minor mistake will lead to undesirable consequences. Here we can say that the rights of individuals are merely likely to be violated when active Euthanasia is illegal, rather than when it is permitted. Now if euthanasia is legalized even then there are serious problems about how to implement the legalization of euthanasia, should there be no laws at all concerning euthanasia ? And if so, then it surely would lead to significant abuse. But if there is need to be laws, what form should they take? If the laws introduced are complex and stringent procedures, then relatively few people who would benefit from euthanasia might wind up being able to do so. On the other hand if the procedures would be very relaxed ones, chances of being misused will increase.

In the end of nineteenth century people began questioning prohibition of euthanasia publicly. The public debate over euthanasia resumed after the 1950s with the development of new life-sustaining technologies such as the mechanical respirator, which has first been used in the 1930s. Along with these advances came a growing concern over the increasing control of technology over life and death. Public opinion began shifting in favour of legalized euthanasia in the early 1970s. As of 1996, 69 per cent of Americans were in favour of permitting doctors to perform euthanasia, if a person has an incurable disease. In a recent 2000 survey of 30,000 Americans over the age of 55, 65 per cent said that people with a terminal illness have the right to hasten their deaths with the assistance of physicians. Support for legalizing euthanasia and physician-assisted suicide tends to be higher in other western countries. Three-quarters of both Canadians and Australians support active euthanasia, including assisted suicide, for terminal illness. 82 per cent of the British would like to see euthanasia, although not necessarily assisted suicides, legalized. Support for euthanasia is especially high in France and in Netherlands where active, voluntary euthanasia has been legal for several years. In China, although euthanasia is illegal, 80 per cent of people surveyed in a1988 poll stated that they were in favour of euthanasia.

Conclusion

In conclusion we can say that in spite of the great diversity of views on this matter we can say that the practice of Euthanasia should be allowed on certain unavoidable and very critical circumstances when all hopes of his or her life has gone off and there remains no other alternatives left. Even in that condition euthanasia should be carried out only by doctors after having full discussions with a group of senior and competent doctors of that field. The doctors should also take into consideration their economical situation and the consent of the patient (if possible) along with the family members must be taken. So the decision to die must be voluntary and considered decision of an informed patient; there must be physical or mental suffering which the sufferer finds unbearable and there is no other reasonable solution to improve the situation. It is the duty of the doctor to do everything possible to try to save the life of the patient but it is not wise to engage in heroic efforts to add another few weeks, days or hours to save the life of a terminally ill and suffering cancer patient or to give active treatment to babies born, so defective that their short life will be filled with little more than continuous suffering.

Mercy for a hopelessly ill and suffering patient and, in the case of voluntary euthanasia, respect for autonomy, have been the primary reasons given by those who have argued for the moral permissibility of euthanasia. Today, there is widespread popular support for some forms of euthanasia and many contemporary philosophers have argued that euthanasia is morally defensible.

Most writers in the field agree that there are times when life-sustaining treatment should be withheld and a patient should be allowed to die. This view is shared even by those who regard euthanasia or the intentional termination of life as always wrong.

Thus, we can say that if practice of euthanasia is permitted we can have lot of potential benefit such as it could be used to prevent the unnecessary prolongation of the suffering experienced by many terminally ill people and their families. We know that there are some kinds of pain which cannot be eliminated with drugs, or at least not with drugs that leave the patient conscious and mentally coherent. And in addition to physical agony, there is often overwhelming emotional suffering for the patient and derivatively for friends and families in attendance. All this can be shortened if euthanasia is allowed.

Another advantage of permitting euthanasia is resource

allocation. The resource, both economic and human, that are now devoted to keeping alive people who have incurable and debilitating diseases can often be more cost-effectively be devoted to curing people of curable diseases, or to funding preventive medicine, or even just to feed the starving. In this way we can say that yes Euthanasia should be permitted and legalized but of course, the law allowing euthanasia should be very well drafted and that law would have to be rigorously policed to prevent misuse.

REFERENCES

1. *A Companion to Applied Ethics*, Edited by R.G.Frey and Christopher Health Wellman.
2. *Ethics in Practice*; An Analogy, Edited by Hugh LaFollette.
3. *Contemporary Issues in Bioethics*, Edited with Introduction, by Tom L. Beauchamp and LeRoy Walters.
4. *Contemporary Debates in Applied Ethics*, Edited by Andrew I. Cohen and Christopher Health Wellman.
5. *Analyzing Moral Issues*, Edited by Judith A. Boss.
6. *Bioethics in a Liberal Society*, Edited by Max Charlesworth.
7. *Applied Ethics*: A Non-Consequentialist Approach, Edited by David S. Oderberg.

Chapter 20

No Flesh Eating Buddhist Perspective of Vegetarianism

A.K. Srivastava

This chapter involves some complex ethical principles that have been discussed down the ages. But before we enter into these complex problems and explain out some difficult knots in this connection, it seems proper to define the term '*vegetarianism*' itself and its importance in the present world. Broadly, the term "*vegetarianism*" means "to support one's life on grain, fruit, milk, cereals, and vegetable only and not to take flesh in any form, in any case." In the contemporary world, the need for vegetarian food is emphasized for two simple reasons. One is pragmatic and second is moral. Even the second moral consideration, is sought to support the first one. Hence, the pragmatic reason is more important. In fact, due to over-dependence on flesh food for taste and good health, the merciless killing of animals in huge quantity, for thousands of years, have caused a great threat to our ecology. There is a possibility that a few birds and a few species of animals may become extinct and create a great threat to our environment that may tell upon us adversely. This is the reason that the warning against killing of birds and animals are given regularly by environmentalists, social institutions and religious leaders and now, by the governments also. Some governments have made killing of certain species of birds and animals a punishable offence. In several States hunting is a punishable offence. The glaring example is of Salman Khan, a film star, who is facing a criminal trial for killing a black deer (Chinkara) in Rajasthan's national sanctuary.

The second pragmatic reason is of human health and hygiene. It is evident from some incidents of recent past, that regular flesh eating is causing a lot of diseases. Physicians have started prescribing vegetarian diet and are propagating the benefits of vegetarian meals. The Yoga Gurus are giving warning against flesh food and are demonstrating its fatality and bad effects. Some have tried to prove it scientifically, that vegetarian foods are in no way inferior in comparison to non-vegetarian one; rather some grains like soya, barley and many others are superior in nutrition than meat, fish and egg. Comparative charts are also available that demonstrate the superiority of vegetarian meals over the non-vegetarian one. An advertisement for using milk regularly is seen on the television screen off and on.

The third pragmatic reason is that, in the recent past, a few people have died and many fell ill after eating red meat. Animal diseases like bird flu, cow fever, infection in beef, and many others have created panicky among the flesh eaters. Now many of them are becoming vegetarian under compulsion, under the fear of deadly diseases. It is a widely accepted fact that normally, we observe any moral precept for two reasons, prize and punishment. In this instance the second alternative, the punishment, in terms of several diseases born out of non-vegetarian foods have forced men to become vegetarian. The social religious and moral activists have come in support of vegetarianism. Slogans like, 'Be vegetarian', Have compassion for animals, 'Animals do have the right to live like you', '*Jiyo aur Jeene do*' are found written on walls in bold letters. Now the time has come to contemplate on this problem seriously. The present discussion is a humble effort in this direction, wherein we will try to investigate into the history of Buddhism, ranging up to 600 B.C. and see, what is the opinion of the Buddha and Buddhism on this subject directly or indirectly.

We have intentionally omitted some of the investigations into the history of vegetarianism, because in this regard no sound inference as to the modern social problems can possibly by drawn from any record of the past. It is interesting to know that Buddha and Mahavira prescribed non-violence and asked the common mass to live on vegetarian diet, but how far their words remained effective in the past and will be in time to come is the problem. They might have been, but yet no one has recorded the effect of their words. This might have been the case, that they spoke for vegetarianism at first by dismay at the sight of great excess in flesh food. It is a fact that Buddha raised His voice against slaughtering of cattle in the *yajna* by Brahmins in the name of sacrifice[1], but there is hardly any evidence of vegetarian practice in mass scale. If there were any, it is difficult to connect it securely with its gradual declining tendency. To be brief, the important question has been, not the practice of vegetarianism by an exceptional minority, but that of the mass of the population—just the large complex fact—which has never been recorded[2]. This is the reason that we do not intend to discuss the history of vegetarianism, rather we expect to discuss some principal aspects of the problem to be considered. They are physiological and ethical aspects.

1. The Physiological Aspect

The physiological argument in favour of vegetarianism is treated as of subordinate importance. The reason is that the evidence gathered in its support from the factual world is incomplete, as it deals with the physiological effects of flesh or non-flesh diet on human mind and body. But it is very difficult to ascertain such effects and arrive at any scientific conclusion, as those experiments have to be conducted under conditions that cannot be obtained in ordinary life. It is impossible to ascertain that any two sets of experiments deals with the same data. In other words, we cannot make it sure that up to what extent mind can influence body in any given circumstances. We cannot say with certainty that any given case has the influence of mind on bodily tissues. It is a fact that vegetarians have provided wonderful records of endurance who take fruits, milk, grains and vegetable only, as well as the prolonged effects of vegetarian diet on mind and muscles.

But it is quite uncertain that whether the spirit of individual in question has not affected the result. Again we have observed that the effect of the vegetarian diet on fair number of individuals and found their health well maintained. However, it is again open for skeptics to insist that for a sound and valid scientific conclusion, the experiment of at least three coming generation is required as in doing so the experiment can be had in different situations. Again vegetarian diet varies from place to place, time-to-time and person-to-person. To ascertain the effects of all the vegetarian diets is not possible. Here another problem arises that the very question of vegetarianism and its experiment is obscured by the variety of diet comprised under the title of 'vegetarian'. Large numbers of people abstain from meat but not from fish. Some take non-vegetarian diet once a week or in a month. Other eat egg neither meat nor fish and so on. To investigate such types of facts in the antiquities of Buddhism would be an utter foolishness. Because of such complexities, neither Buddha nor his disciples ever made such experiments or intended to do so. The reason is simple; their purpose was not to advocate vegetarianism, as it was not the demand of tho day. But it is again the fact that Buddha asked his followers to abstain from non-vegetarian diet as far as possible, because vegetarian foods have positive effects on their thought and action. At one place he has categorically said, "Those who eat *samaka*, *kingulaka*, and *kanika*, *pattaphala*, *mulaphala*, and *gariphala* (different sorts of grass, leafs, roots, etc.) justly obtained by the just, do not speak falsehood (nor are they) desirous of sensual pleasure[3]. He further adds. "He who eats what has been well prepared, well dressed, what pure and excellent, given others, he who enjoys food made of rice, meat, O Kassapa nothing defiles him"[4]. These two verses of Suttanipata's *Amgandha Sutta* hints, directly or indirectly, that even though such experiments were not made by Buddha to his disciples in connection with vegetarian diet, even then He was of the view that food influence the thought and action of a person. Vegetarian foods have positive and soothing effects on human behaviour as well as it keeps one away from defilements. However, it was not the principal problem for Buddha, it was not his main concern to prescribe vegetarian diet and advocate for it, rather his fight was against *dukkha samudaya*, of which human is grappled internally and externally[4]. His sole purpose was to eradicate it. However, some references are available wherein we find that Buddhist kings have passed orders to abstain from flesh eating. King Ashoka, after embracing Buddhism, passed an order to abstain from flesh eating on a particular day. He made laws against animal killing on observance day. He also banned indiscriminate burning the forest, castrating and branding of cattle. Not only this, some Theravada kings have also prohibited and delimited the slaughter of animals. But this does not mean that they were vegetarians and they were propagating vegetarianism or its values. On the contrary, Buddha himself seems to have accepted meat in his alms-bowl. It is evident from *Mahaparinibbana Sutta* that Buddha has eaten meat before his death (*parinibbana*). Rather, it is said that the immediate cause of his physical death was eating pork (*sukaramaddava*) offered by Cund-kammaraputta, a goldsmith. In fact, after eating the meat he became the victim of acute blood dysentery, which caused his death[5]. The above discussion categorically indicate that the physiological aspect of vegetarianism is completely lacking in early or in later Buddhism, hence, there is no need to carry on any investigation in this regard in Buddhist context.

2. The Ethical Aspect

This aspect of vegetarianism is more important. It can be appreciated in the light of Buddhist moral approach. In this connection the first precept of Buddha, not to kill or abstain from violence (*panatipata veramani*) becomes very important. It is a resolution not to kill or injure any human, animal, bird, fish or insect. The fifth step of *astanga marga*, prescribed by Buddha, the Right Livelihood (*Samma Ajiva*) is again very important. It asks one not to support one's life through wrong means and one of the wrong means is trading in flesh. If both the precepts are observed in a proper way, it will give rise to vegetarian practices in the common mass as killing and trading in flesh both are sins. Buddhists are supposed to adhere to the first precept (to abstain from killing) and observe the Right Livelihood (*Samma Ajiva*) properly. This will generate a vegetarian feeling in individuals and vegetarianism will find its proper place in the society.

Here a question arises, will simply preaching non-violence or chanting repeatedly *panatipata veramani* or observe Right Livelihood (samma ajiva), inculcate vegetarian culture in the society? Certainly, it is not so. It may affect the exceptional minority but not the populace at large. The question is how to generate this feeling in human mind? What should be the *modus operandi* to make the people at least think in terms of vegetarian diet? In order to arrive at the ways and means to generate vegetarian feeling in humankind, this needs to be discussed in the light of three points of views, as this problem has three aspects. They are utilitarian, sociological and moral. A brief discussion of all the three is desirable here.

(i) Utilitarian Perspective

Utilitarianism is an ethical theory, which believes in 'greatest good in greatest number'. Buddha too, talks of *bahujana hitaya bahujana sukhaya*, i.e., benefit of many, and pleasure of many. Hence, while deciding any course of action or prescribing any concept or precept the benefit, pleasure and opinion of majority of the common people have to be taken into consideration. While talking about vegetarianism, we must take into consideration three things; (a) Benefits of vegetarian diet in comparison to the flesh food; (b) taste and preference of the mass with regard to the above mentioned two types of food; and (c) the suitability of the alternative opinion. Let us discuss them one by one.

(a) Benefits of the Vegetarian Diet in comparison to the Non-vegetarian one : It is a common belief that eggs, meat, and fish are

qualitatively greater in nutrition than fruits, cereals, and milk. This is the reason that people opt flesh eating as it provides greater strength and vigour. Earlier physicians also prescribed meat, fish and egg for physically weak persons or who have recuperated from long ailment. And if somehow one could prove that flesh foods are indispensable for one's existence, of course there would be nothing to be said in favour of vegetarianism. If such foods maintain one's health in a better way in comparison to the other one, he has right to eat it. But it has been said earlier that these contentions cannot be verified. On the contrary a large number of population are living with vigour that are taking fruits and herbs for many generations. Such are the examples of Jains, Vaishnavas and a few others in India. Hence, the plea of necessity of taking flesh food for strength and vigour breaks down in the presence of the admitted facts. Now we can in no way defend killing of animals for our selfish ends. In the light of the above-mentioned facts it becomes apparent that one can maintain equally good health and live with vigour even if one spares flesh food (meat eating). This proves that man's whole attitude towards the animal-kingdom is vitiated by selfishness, which is unethical too. Buddha's statement regarding persons maintaining his life on vegetarian diet is the testimony to the fact that such persons not only lead a healthy life but also are pious from within[6]. In such a situation the Utilitarian's argument in favour of meat eating falls flat, rather it supports the vegetarian's contention.

(b) Taste and Preference of the Mass: An empirical study in this connection reveals the fact that minority of the human population accepts the benefits of the vegetarianism as well as welfare of animals. Minority is of the opinion that slaughtering the animals should be condemned only because flesh foods are not preferable, as certain amount of inconvenience would be caused by the change of diet. Here, we face an ethical dilemma. If greatest good in greatest number is the yardstick of morality to implement vegetarianism in strict sense of the term, it will violate the general conscience, if not, the daily commission of slaughtering the animals would be a moral sin. Further the public opinion on the matter of

butchering the animals is too lax as well as the custom is too strong to allow to discuss this issue fairly well, as in the name of religious sacraments or rituals animals are being slaughtered or sacrificed. In this way the majority of human population is too much under the yoke of religio-social customs to raise a human appeal against the heinous crime against the animals. The parameter of the mass opinion and the pleasure of many find support from western moral thinkers. J.S. Mills is of the opinion that each person's happiness is good to that person and the general happiness is, therefore, good to the aggregate of all persons. He further opines that it is quite compatible with the principles of utility to recognize the fact that some type of pleasure is more desirable and valuable than others. And since majority of the population prefer the taste of non-vegetarian meals in comparison to the vegetarian one, one is helpless to argue in favour of vegetarianism. The reason is that out of the two pleasures, if there is one who have experienced the both, give express preference, irrespective of any feeling of moral obligation to prefer it, that is desirable pleasure. In such a situation vegetarian's argument succumbs to the heavy pressure of the meat eaters. This argument may get support of Aristippus, Helvetious, Bentham and many others in the west and Carvaka in India.

(c) The Suitability of the Alternative Option : Whether vegetarian food is a suitable option for the meat eaters or not, is again a controversial issue. What should be the measuring rod for suitability is yet to be decided. But in common use, suitability may broadly mean usefulness. Here usefulness means useful to the health or at least equally good impact on mind and body. The comparative charts of the nutrition value of both the foods (vegetarian and non-vegetarian) reveal the fact that fruits, milk, cereals and herbs are in no way inferior to the flesh food. In some cases these are superior. It has been scientifically demonstrated that milk, cereals (grains), fruits, etc., are sufficient to support the human life in full vigour. Buddha is also of the opinion that vegetarian foods are effective in producing healthy effect on human body as well as it keeps the mind happy and pure. "He who hopes for fruits, cultivates energy that produces joy and pleasure that

brings praise while carrying the human yoke[7] On the basis of the above discussion it can be said that vegetarian diet can supplant the non-vegetarian one. As long as there is a reason to believe that animal flesh is no better (indeed is inferior) as food for men as fruits and vegetables, it cannot be right to kill the animal and eat them[8].

In the light of the above discussion if we cast our glance over Buddha's life, Buddhist thought and literature, we do not find any support of vegetarianism as is found in modern thoughts. It is a fact that Buddha preached non-violence (*panatipata veramani*) and asked one to adhere to the right livelihood (*sammajiva*) in a proper way and in right spirit but these also cannot support the vegetarian cause. The basic reason is he did not observe vegetarianism in strict sense of the term. On the contrary at several places, he rated meat eating morally greater than some evils or unholy deeds. In *Suttanipata,* he says, "The charge of defilement (*amagandha*) does not apply to me, 'so thou sayest O' Brahman, enjoying food (made) of rice together with well prepared bird flesh[9]." He further narrates a number of impurities and impure activities, such as greed, hatred, obstinacy, bigotry, deceit and very many traits to which flesh eating is morally better[10]. These words directly or indirectly weakens the vegetarian cause and vegetarian's arguments, even if these do not promote meat eating. We scare that someone may utilize these *Buddhavacana* in nursing their greed of flesh eating while this was not the intention of the Buddha.

(ii) Sociological Perspective

Sociology, to my mind, deals with human behaviour and social relations, mobility and change in ordinary business of life. When a life style is changed, it studies its pros and cons in terms of sociological implications as even a small change in the taste and habit of human beings causes a great change in employment or unemployment at the state and global level. Taking into consideration these facts and fiction, the meat eaters may argue that, "If abstinence from meat becomes general, intolerable evil would result, such as the means of livelihood would be taken from millions of workers. There will be loss of skin which are needed for clothing and which are supplied, at present, from animal's breed[11]." If vegetarian diet is implemented strictly, or if people in large number change their food habit from meat to fruit, cereal, vegetable and milk, a chaotic situation may emerge as a large number of big or small industries trading in flesh or in animal products will be destroyed and millions of workers will be thrown out of employment. We can easily understand the plight of their dependents. From humanitarian point of view, vegetarianism cannot be advocated as it may result in gross unemployment and render the workers of leather and meat industries jobless.

Above argument is based on two misconceptions or wrong assumptions. The first is that the propagation of vegetarianism will cause a vast revolution in diet because of sudden arrangement. Secondly, there is no suitable potential industry in other sector that may provide an alternative arrangement in terms of mass employment. However, there is no reason to assume anything of this kind at least in all those countries where conservative prejudices on this subject is adamantine In fact, the results of conduct in this case is far too uncertain to be worth arguing about. Nor in this case there is any need to forecast the future with laborious precision, which is often effected. In fact, even in the Buddhist country a few Buddhists are meat eater. In such a case the assumption of switching over to vegetarian meals in mass scale out of sudden is ridiculous and untenable. Secondly even if, miraculously, this change takes place there is nothing to worry about. Industrialization and expansion of business in a massive way have created a number of alternative job opportunities in modern world. In such a situation, the Right Livelihood (*sammajiva*) prescribed by the Buddha as the fifth step of His Eight Fold Path, can be observed very easily. In the Right Livelihood, the Buddha has ruled out trade in flesh. He has condemned butchers, hunters and fishermen only because as a profession they do not observe the first precept, abstinence from violence (*panatipataveramani*). Since these professions are based on violence (*himsa* or *panatipata*) no committed Buddhist can carry on these jobs. The butchers are usually non-Buddhists, mostly Muslims, and they are considered outcaste and seen as deprived. Buddhist countries lack mass slaughterhouses, as it is seen in the West. These things are seen as hell on the earth. This is the reason Buddhists do not raise livestock for slaughter, as it is seen as breach of Right Livelihood which they tend to steer clear off[12].

Secondly, in the modern world the relation between man and the animal is based on the logic of domination. It is a well-known fact that from the point of view of ecology man and animal both are the members of the biotic community. It is again considered that man is on so much higher a plane that he has the ability to effect, influence, change and modify the nature and natural entities as per his needs and specification. In his design and utility he can use the things and beings of the nature. Whosoever is capable to change is superior and whatever gets changed is inferior to him. And whosoever is superior has the right to dominate the other. Now in such a situation human welfare must get precedence in all the cases. Since flesh is essential for good health and vigour of man he has the right to kill and eat animals. This argument, however, may look sound and lucrative from man's point of view, but in the Buddhist context, this logic runs in a different way. In place of '*Logic of Domination*' here we find the '*Logic of Compassion*'. According to this logic, man is the highest (not the best) evolutes of nature. At the same time this placement as the 'Highest Evolute' has also given him the responsibility to protect and promote the entire cosmic existence[13], including the animals and not to kill them due to greed, hatred an delusion. The logic behind this is that the superiors have the duty to protect and extend loving kindness to the subordinates and the inferiors. Just as the mother protects her child at the cost of her own life, in the same way, one must have loving kindness towards all beings of the world and human heart must get saturated with motherly affection for other beings too.[14] In the same spirit Buddha says, "may all beings be happy and secure... whatever living beings there are ... feeble and strong, long, short or medium, small or large... may all beings, without exception, be happy minded[15]. If one's thinking is regulated by the Buddha's

Logic of compassion, one's vision towards the animal kingdom will be transformed and a paradigm shift may take place between their relations. Now both are the members of the same biotic family, hence relation between them will be of protector and to be protected instead of means and end. In such a situation one will never like to kill and eat animals for one's selfish ends (taste and health) and it will be easier to become vegetarian. However, the appeal to human compassion in matters of treatment to animals and turning towards the vegetarian diet, though logically cogent, has made a little success even in the country where the sentiment of kindness toward animals is strongly developed. One of the reasons behind it is the chasm between the precept and practice, thought and action and preaching and behaviour of the followers of even the champions of non-violence (*ahimsa*). This controversy needs to be discussed under ethico-moral aspect of the problem in hand.

(iii) The Moral Aspect

If man recognizes the claim of animals to good treatment, then the situation may change. But the result of the opposite line of conduct is not easy to see. And this is the point where the religious considerations supplement ethical. If we believe that the animals have been committed to us, we are bound to treat them kindly even if the results were likely to be far more inconvenient than they possibly could be. But the controversy arises when we find that the Buddha himself has partaken of animal food and the immediate cause of his death was eating the pork. In such a situation how can an earthly creature take a firm stand on His first precept of non-violence? How can an ignorant man, who is in the state of bondage, check his temptation of eating meat as well as becoming firm on His first precept of non-violence and abstain from killing (*panatipatapata veramani*)? And this controversy regarding the problem in hand, Vegetarianism and Buddhism, takes a different turn. Now the question does not remain here whether Buddha preached, prescribed or consented to vegetarianism or not. Rather the question here is that under what circumstances Buddha partook flesh food and how can we rationalize the two contradictory practices, preaching non-violence and eating meat? How can this chasm of precept and practice be bridged, with regard to the Buddha and Buddhist monks? With regard to these questions and queries, it can be said that any of the teachings of the Buddha cannot be quoted in favour of slaying animals for eating meat. But at the same time it appears quite legitimate to argue that He has no objection to this practice on humanitarian ground. Here two points seem very important to be discussed. (1) Why is there a chasm between precept and practice? (2) What are the grounds or what type of meat Buddha allowed eating? Here we will discuss the second query first.

It has already been discussed earlier that Buddha denounced killing and asked not to harm any living being[16] but surprisingly He was not against meat eating. Rather He allowed Bikkhus to accept what has been put in their alms-bowl[17], as purity does not depend on the food only, but also on the mental state and right food vision[18]. In *Majjhima Nikaya*, He has prescribed the rules regarding meat eating. In the *Jivaka Sutta* under the heading of the '*Tikotiparsuddham Mansani*' He has said that in three cases one cannot use the meat, if it is seen, heard, and suspected to have killed for the purpose of a monk[19]. Because such meat is blemished. But if it is not seen, not heard and not even suspected to have been killed for a monk's purpose, then only a monk can eat it, provided it is given to him in his alms-bowl, as such meat is unblemished. This is how He meets with or replies the allegation of meat eating[20]. Perhaps this is the reason Buddha does not find any sin to a monk, if some acquires meat for him. At the same time, Buddha also warns that whosoever intentionally prepares meat for Tathagata and Bhikkhus, or orders to kill the animal, or brings the animal forcefully on the slaughter place and places before monks the above mentioned prepared meat accrues a great sin. The cry of the animal, because of pain, during slaying it, also accumulates a great sin for the persons who have been instrumental in killing it for food.

Buddha has allowed using animal flesh, blood, and oil in case of sickness or ailment in form of medicine. He say, "I allow, O

Bhikkhus, in case of disease ... the use of raw flesh and blood[21]. Cooking and eating of the remains of the kills of the lion, hyenas and wolves have also been allowed to the Bhikkhus[22]. However, Buddha has prohibited the monks to use the meat of ten animals for various reasons[23]. They are man, elephant, horse, dog, snake, lion, tiger, leopard, bear and hyena. In the light of above-mentioned facts it can be said that the Early Buddhist attitude towards meat eating and Buddha's first precept of non-violence appears to be contradictory.

It is interesting to note that a few Mahayanies disagree with the Theravadins on the point that the Buddha allowed the Bhikkhus to eat meat under certain circumstances. *Lankavatarasutra*, a text of Mahayana tradition, denies that the Buddha has allowed blameless meat for monks. It argues against meat eating in this way : "All beings have relatives in the past life ... meat stinks; eating it hinders meditation and leads to a bad health, arrogance and rebirth as a carnivorous animals or low class human. If meat is not eaten, killing for consumption will cease"[24]. Peter Harvey is of the opinion that "In China, the first precept (or at least the *Boddhisattva* vows) has been seen as entailing vegetarianism, so that monks, nuns and pious lay devotees have avoided meat, and vegetarian foods have been common at Buddhist celebrations. In Japanese tradition, no beef has been eaten and vegetarianism has existed, especially among Zen monks"[25].

Conclusion

The above discussions lead to the conclusion that Buddha neither prescribed vegetarianism nor recommended flesh eating in the strict sense of the term. No such references are available in the Pali canons wherein either vegetarianism or non-vegatarianism have been recommended or forbidden by Him. The reason is very simple. The question regarding diet was not a burning problem of that time as is found in our age. But for arriving at any conclusion regarding these in Buddhist context, one will have to keep into consideration the trends of thoughts that were prevalent before and during the Buddha's time as Buddha was not unaware of the long tradition of history. Preceding Him there were two schools of thoughts. One believed in living eats living (*jiva jivasya bhojanam*) and cattle offering in the *yajana* is not violence at all. (*Vediki himsa himsa na bhavati*). These directly or indirectly encouraged flesh eating, as these provided a religious sanction for killing, castrating and maiming animals, birds, and other living objects for being served as delicious and healthy dishes both for the affluent and the laity. The other school strictly adhered to the dictum '*ahimsa paramo dharmah*' this means 'non-violence is the supreme religion' or 'in non-violence lies the essence of the religion'. This lays stress on eating fruit, milk, and cereals by altogether rejecting flesh food in any form or kind. Buddha, being a Middle Path holder had to strike a balance between the two. It was more than urgent because Buddha was not only a recluse saint or a spiritualist; He was a social reformer as well. To achieve His purpose He preached moderation in all walks of life. He felt with conviction that mankind could relieve himself from the yoke of *dukkha* (persecution) by adopting the 'Middle Path' (*madhyam marga*) in action and spirit. Hence, He was compelled to survey the demographic map of human habit and taste. The majority appeared to be in favour of flesh eating whereas a perceptible section favoured vegetarianism. Olden religious rites even encouraged through *yajana, havana* and sacrificed animals on festive occasions and worship of different deities. In such a situation Buddha could not have gone altogether in opposing column. In that case His very purpose of social reformation could have ended in fiasco. So to strike balance and maintain social coherence. He dwelt strongly on rejection of flesh-eating showing its manifold advantages both on physical and spiritual levels but allowed restricted flesh-eating on physical (like illness), climatic (like extremely cold region) and economic (like abject poverty) grounds. This was in tune of His life philosophy which can be summed up as "*bahujana hitaya bahujana sukhaya*", that is for the happiness and comfort of the maximum.

REFERENCES

1. It is evident from Payasi, Sutta that Kassapa, a prominent disciple of the Buddha denounced the killing of animals in the name of sacrifice in *yajna.* He says, "At the sort of sacrifice, Prince, where oxen are slain, or goats, or fowls and pigs or diverse creatures are put to an end; and those who take part in the sacrifice have wrong views, wrong intention, wrong speech, wrong action, wrong livelihood, wrong endeavour, wrong mindfulness, and wrong rapture. Such sacrifices, O Prince, is neither of great fruitlessness nor of a great profit, nor of great renown, nor of widespread effect. Is just as if a farmer, prince, were to enter a wood taking with him plough and seed, and were there, in an untilted tract, in unfavourable soil, among uprooted sumps, to plant seeds that were broken, rotten, spoilt by wind and heat out of season, not in good condition, and gods were not to give rain in due season. *Digh Nikaya* II 351-53; The translation is taken from the *Dialogues of the Buddha*, II, *pp.* 370-71 (Translated by Rhys Davids). Low Price Publication, Delhi, First Published In 1910, reprinted in 2000.
2. *Encyclopedia of Religion and Ethics*, Vol. 12, Edit. James Hastings, Edinburgh: T and T Clark and New York Charles, Scribner's Sons 5th impression, pp. 618-19.
3. *Suttanipata, Amagandhasutta, Gutha* No. 1 (238); The translation is taken from *Sacred Book of the East.* (S.B.E.) Vol. X, Part-II, Trans. Maxmullar, Motilal Banarsidas, Delhi, 1965, Reprint 1998, p. 39.
4. *Anto jata bahi jata, jataye jatita paja. Samayutta Nikaya Jata Sutta; Visuddhimaggo* Vol. I.
5. "*Evam, bhante,ti kho cundakammaroputto bagvato patisuttvayam ahosi sukarmaddavam patiyattam tena bhagavantam parivisi; ..Ath kho bhagavato cunddassa kammarputtass battam buttavissa kharo abadho uppajji.... Lohitapakkhandika paballahvedana vattantimara-nantiki. Digha Nikaya*, Vol. II, *Mahaparinibbanasutta*, 127, 127.
6. *Suttanipata, Amagandhasutta. Gatha* 2 (139) The translation is taken from *Sacred Book of the East,* (S.B.E.), Vol. X.
7. *Ibid., Hirisutta, Gatha* 4 (255) *Sacred Book of the East,* (S.B.E.), Vol. X, part-II, p. 42.
8. *Encyclopaedia of Religion and Ethics*, Vol. 12, *op.cit.*, p. 620.
9. *Suttanipata, Amagandhasutta. Gatha* no. 3; The translation is taken from *Sacred Book of the East*, (S.B.E.), Vol. X, Part-II, p. 39.
10. *Ibid., Gutha* No. 4-10 (241-47).

11. *Encyclopaedia of Religion and Ethics*, Vol. 12, *op. cit.*, p. 620.
12. *An Introduction to Buddhism*, Peter Harey, Munshiram Manoharlal Publishers Pvt. Ltd., Delhi, 1990, pp. 203-4.
13. Avinash Kumar Srivastava, *Buddhist Environmentalism, Readings in Environmental Ethics*, Rawat Publication, Jaipur, Delhi, 2005, pp. 144.
14. *Mata yatha niyam puttamayusaekaputtamanurakkhe Evam hi sabbabhutesu, manasam bhavaye aparimanam.....Khuddakapath, Mettasutta, Gatha* 7.
15. *Ye keci panbhutatthi, tasa va thavara vanasa.....Digha va ye va mahanta majjhimarasska anukathuta. Dittha va ye va adittha sabbasattabhavantusukhinah. Ibid.*, Gutha No. 4, 5.
16. *Pano na hantabbo.....Digha Nikaya*, II, 173-74.
17. *Sacred Book of the East*, Vol. XIII, *op.cit*, p. 155.
18. *Yato aharasamudayanirodham pajanati.... Majjhima Nikaya,* Vol. I, pp. 47-49.
19. *Tihi kho aham, jivaka, thanehi, mansam paribhogani, ti vadami. Afittham, asutam, aparisankitam-imehikhoaham, jivaka, tihi thanehi mansamparibhogamti vadama. Majjhima Nikaya*, Vol. I, p. 49.
20. *Ibid.*, pp. 368-71.
21. *Sacred Book of the East*, Vol. XVII, *op. cit.*, p. 49.
22. *Ibid.*, Vol. XVII, p. 43.
23. *Ibid.*, Vo. XVIV, pp. 85-86.
24. *Lankaatarasutra*, 244-59; quoted in *An Introduction to Buddhism, op.cit.*, p. 204.
25. *An Introduction to Buddhism, op.cit.*, p. 204.

Chapter 21

Bioethical Concerns in Hinduism

Madhumita Chatterjee

Broadly speaking the discipline which deals with the challenging issues arising from medical practices and biological researches, different Life Sciences is termed bioethics in the west. Some of the major issues which come under the purview of bioethics are euthanasia, *in vitro* fertilization, *cloning, stem-cell therapy, organ transplantation, genetic engineering, suicide, abortion and others.* Ethical disputes that arise regarding these issues are : what should be the role of medical practitioners, clinicians and patients particularly in cases of euthanasia, organ transplantation, abortion, *in vitro* fertilization and others. In all these cases, question arises what exactly constitute the sphere of the authority of the patients, physicians and others? To what extent should these various clinical and medical practices be kept confidential from the public? How far the government should intervene and regulate and control such researches? Whether the medical practitioners and researchers have ethical responsibilities to disclose their activities to the common people. How much autonomy should be given to the decision of the patients in these cases and many other questions.

The term 'bioethics' was first coined in the early 1970s to discuss the aforesaid issues. By 1980, many medical schools all over Europe arranged programmes and journals to discuss these challenging issues and find out the path for resolution. Within 2000 bioethics became an internationally recognized, interdisciplinary discipline including philosophers, medical practitioners, biologists, ethnologists as well as historians within its ambience. Thinkers from different perspectives often disagree with each other. Some bioethicists want to confine ethical evaluation of actions (mainly medical treatments and sophisticated biological research) that might help or harm only human beings. Other intend to widen the scope of ethical evaluation to include the morality of actions that might help or harm all organisms, who have sensitivity, are able to feel pleasure and pain, and include these actions within the scope of bioethics, if they are related to medicine and biology. Bioethicists inspite of their difference of opinion, want to discuss and solve the aforesaid problems honestly and intelligently using insights and observations from other disciplines. Cardinal principles which are acknowledged to be the foundation of biomedical and behavioural researches mainly involving human beings, are autonomy, beneficence and justice. These principles are also being tried to be extended to other creatures by some thinkers. Non-malfeasance, or non-injury, human dignity and sanctity of life are also the latest additions to the aforesaid list of ethical principles. The development of bioethics as an independent academic discipline and a flourishing industry is a recent phenomenon, although discussions about different moral issues, were present in medicine in the west since the ancient time of Hippocratic oath, where not to harm was prescribed for the medical practitioners.

Unlike Western tradition, Hinduism did not have any systematically arranged, separate academic and articulate discipline called bioethics. which we call in the present day. Hinduism in its own way saw life and its problems and sufferings and we see that even in such an ancient period Hinduism believed in the principles like sanctity of life, respect for all life, autonomy and dignity of an individual which are considered to be the basic ethical principles used to solve dilemmas, we face in bioethics and controversies in the present century. These above mentioned principles are perhaps universal principles which do not remain confined to any time and place. Hinduism had a culture where religion, medicine and ethics made a common entry to each other's periphery. In fact they were intimately related to each other to build up a total discipline.

All ideas of Hinduism regarding Euthanasia, abortion, sucicide, cloning, organ transplantation, genetic engineering follow from their close link between humans and the entire nature as well as their views on suffering, life and death, the theory of *Karma*, cosmology and transmigration of souls. The way they looked and faced these problems denote that these problems were also present since ancient time and perhaps their way of solving such controversies regarding these matters may help us to throw some light on recent bioethical problems. Now I shall try to concentrate my discussions on the different issues of the Hindu views on euthanasia, suicide, abortion, organ-transplantation, *in vitro* fertilization, surrogate motherhood and other issues as well as a brief account on Hindu medicine in general.

Regarding Hinduism we must start our discussion by saying that Hinduism believed suffering to be an unavoidable reality of life. Suffering includes both mental and physical suffering. To get freedom from physical suffering, Hinduism developed its own way to maintain good health, to cure illlness and wanted to delay mortal death, by reducing the sufferings associated with it. For these reasons Hinduism developed a very elaborate and advanced system of medicine, a glimpse of which we find in Ayurveda. *Moksha* was considered to be the highest ideal to a Hindu which meant freedom from all sufferings physical and mental forever. The ideal of *moksha* or Liberation was not only a theoretical concept but it was prescribed in practical life as well. Leading a virtuous life through right conduct would help one to progress gradually towards the ideal. Hindus practiced what they preached. In order to remove the physical suffering. We shall now discuss the nature of Hindu medicine, health, disease and morality. Hinduism shares positive attitude towards medicine as well as the art of healing.

Ayurveda was a complex, and elaborate medical system which was developed in India over the first millennium B.C. According to Ayurveda, health and disease is based on the balance of three substances or *dosas*, namely wind (*vata*), bile (*pitta*) and phlegm (*kapha*). Excess of one over others and their locus in the body determines the nature of particular diseases — physical and mental, and their symptoms. To cure a disease, a physician is to restore, the balance between these three elements, mentioned before, with the help of medicine diet, massage, purification and giving directions to the diseased, to lead an appropriate life-style.[1] Ayurveda, also rcognized other external causes that provided a better account than humoral imbalance to explain medical conditions of the patient. The theory of *Karma* played a prominent role here. Illness or any deformity might be caused by the sins committed in previous births, for example, a person born with a deformed hand could be said to have done a misdeed in his or her previous lives. This condition however, did not discourage efforts on the part of the patient to improve his condition by surgery. Since the duration of punishment through *karma* was unknown and the trouble might be only temporary. Moreover unethical behaviour and violent actions of conduct in one's present life were not confined to effect on that individual but they could have a grave effect on the future generation as well. Even if a king committed misdeeds, it might produce epidemic diseases and disasters. There were other factors besides *Karma* which promoted health or disease. Devotion to God might also promote longevity and health, to the devotee[2] Now I shall try to concentrate my discussion on the major issues of Hindu bioethics.

Broadly speaking in acient India three basic types of death are recognized i.e., natural, unnatural (eing killed) and self willed (killing oneself) The category of self willed death included three different types—suicide, voluntary death and religious self willed death.

Euthanasia may be the first object of our study. Euthanasia is a phenomenon where one voluntarily destroys one's own body for several reasons. Such self destruction is considered to be a bad *karma* in Hindu view. When an individual undergoes intolerable pain and suffering for a long time and selects death for him, rejects any medical help and any care and support by others such an action is not supported by Hinduism. Hinduism wants that persons should die naturally in the course of the biological process. People who are involved in this process of self-annihilation voluntarily according to Hinduism will have to bear the burden of the *Prarabdha Karma* of the dying person proportionately. And people who will provide assistance to such an activity either directly or indirectly cannot escape a similar *Karmic* situation in this life or future life. Euthanasia may be considered to be one type of suicide. Here we come to the idea of suicide in relation to discussions on euthanasia. Suicide in Hindu life is accepted as an act of destruction of life, and an act against humanity. Such deaths are considered to be bad deaths. Suicide was prohibited, since it was self-willed death. These deaths are violent, premature and uncontrollable taking place in wrong place and in wrong time[3]. Suicide is induced by passion depression or uncontrollable circumstances. *Atmaghata* and *atmahatya* became the technical terms for suicide in the late classical period.[4] A person committing suicide in Hindu view is ignorant about the nature of life and human destiny. Such a person will have to continue to remain within the cycle of birth, suffering and death. People who provide assistance to such an action will also face punishment, since the cardinal principle of *ahimsa* has been violated by destruction of life as we have seen in our discussion on euthanasia. But since Hinduism is basically altruistic in nature and, therfore, gives priority to other's welfare so when an individual wants to die for spiritual enlightenment—either for compassion or concern for the welfare of others, such self willed deaths aimed for promoting some greater causes are considered to be good death. These self-willed deaths which may bring spiritual liberation has been known as *prayopravesha* and has been regarded with high esteem. Manu, the first Hindu law giver allowed *prayopravesha* for ascetics, Brahmin and kings. In the case of *prayopravesha*, a person has the freedom to for go medical treatment, to refuse any offered care by family or friends. Viewed for this viewpoint euthanasia or suicide is observed to be an acceptable practice since it promotes one to attain the highest human destiny, i.e., liberation.

Regarding the method of organ transplantation we may now proceed to discuss organ transplantation. For this we have to discuss Hindu process of cremation. Cremation is a very important part of Hindu *samskara*. It is both a destructive process and a process of new creation. After death the physical body of an individual which is constituted of *panch-bhuta* or five natural elements and minds reunite with nature. After the final act of cremation takes place the *atman* continues the *samsara* cycle after wandering for twelve days. So question arises that if the body reunifies with nature without the original set of organs whether the *atman* be allowed to continue *samsara*, and have *karmic* repercussion and take rebirth? This idea about organ transplantation mainly comes from the Hindu idea of transmigration of souls. Many Hindus believe that if the body is incomplete during *samsara*, the dead person's self is suspended in a State of animation and members of the family have to take up *karmic* burden of the dead as a result. No specific religious law forbids organ transplantation and donation of organs. But when one donates an organ for benevolent activities, and when permission is granted such an action accumulates tremendous *karmic* merit and virtue to the donor and would take precedence over organ withdrawn before cremation of the body.[5]

Regarding other issues, like *in vitro* fertilization, transfer of embryo, surrogate motherhood, Hinduism answers in affirmative but it prescribes to practice them only within limits and in accordance to norms and regulations accepted by the society. This is because continuity of life, propagation of species are considered to be the principal tenet of Hindu tradition. Some authors are of the opinion that xenotransplantation may be allowed in Hinduism. It is because respect for different animals can be traced back to the early times of Indus Valley civilization. Animals were not reduced to the status of an object to be used for man's will. Respect which they enjoyed showed a close link between different forms of life in the great chain of life.[6] Regarding cloning, Hindu theory takes an intermediate position. Three principles on which Hindu observations on cloning stands are three principles of nonmalfeasance, beneficence and autonomy. The principle of non-malfeasance is derived from *ahimsa*, a cardinal principle in Hinduism. Viewed from this principle, safety and well-being of the foetus or the potential child is given the prime priority. Premature termination of life is not accepted even if it fosters greater social and scientific welfare of the society. Form the principle of non-malfeasance, Hindu thought concludes that it is not morally justified for science to create a child using somatic cell nuclear transfer cloning because the techniques is not safe for humans.[7] But from the principle of autonomy the above prescription may seem to be otherwise.

Abortion is to be understood to mean a "deliberate termination of pregnancy"[8] In Hinduism the terms generally used for abortion are *garbha-bhruna hatya* or *vadha*.[9] These terms suggest that killing or *hatya* of the foetus has taken place. In classical India, abortion at any stage of pregnancy is not considered to be a morally accepted act, since it disturbs the personal integrity of the unborn. It is because in Hinduism a human being is a complex unit of spirit (*atman*) and matter (*prakriti*). *Atman* is conscious and "actionless, selfdependent, sovereign all —pervading and omnipresent reality which controls body and observe its activities. While physical body or matter is made up of five *mahabhutas* or natural elements."[10] During unison of male and female, the psychic disposition along with the blood is carried to the embryo. So the embryo contains *atman* and *prakriti* within it from the time of conception and killing a foetus who is a sentient being with conscious experience, prematurely violates the cardinal principle of *ahimsa*. So soul in the foetus gets hindrance to the path of salvation not being allowed to take birth and do good *karma*. So it is a grave injustice in Hinduism. Embryo is not the individual concern of mother, But production of offspring is a public duty.[11] Abortion is, however not morally condemned only when the question of preserving mother's life arises. Hindu tradition as we have seen has always accorded personal moral status to the embryo throughout pregnancy.

Last but not the least, we should also mention that what were the duties entrusted to the physicians who were the persons who were directly responsible in handling these cases. It was they who dealt with complicated cases like euthanasia, *in vitro* fertilization, embryo-transfer. Regarding the duty of the physician regarding handling these issues the physicians were advised to possess extensive theoretical knowledge in his field and he should also be honest and practice cleanliness while the patients to be handled were also advised to be obedient and honest, fearless and should provide detailed information about the problems one is suffering from. Physicians are also required to support sick, poor or needy and to treat them with respect. *A vaidya's* religious duty consisted in relieving the suffering of the patients and make them happy. A physician's training in ancient India started with a solemn initiation, where his teacher or *guru* instructed him to lead a frugal and ascetic life, to be a celibate and a vegetarian[12] while undergoing training. He was advised to pray for all beings and must try with all power to heal the sick. He should not betray his patients. Having entered a patient's home, a physician speech, mind and intellect should be devoted to take care of the patients. This oath has been compared to Hippocratic oath of the west. But a physician should refuse to make treatments of the enemies of the kings, women who are unattended by husband or guardian or patients who are about to die. The *vaidya* was advised to look out for new drugs and methods of treatment to enhance knowledge always. In ancient India, the provision of free medical care to the poor was considered as a part of king's duty to protect his subjects. Since the time of Emperor Ashoka, medical clinics of one kind or other, grew up and professional doctors provided free service to the poors. These clinics supported by the states but they were often financed by the private charity.[13]

REFERENCES

1. Weiss, Mitchel, G "Bioethics in Hinduism" in *Encyclopaedia of Bioethics* (Ed) by post Stephen. G. pub. by Thoson Gale, 2004, p. 1145.
2. *Ibid.*

3. Young Katherine K, "*Euthanasia in Hindu Ethics*" *in purity, abortion and euthanasia* by Harold G. Coward, Julius J. Lipner, Katherine K. Young, Pub. by State University of New York Press, p. 74.
4. *Ibid*., p. 75.
5. An article adapted from student bmj- shaheen. lakhan
6. Cromwell. Crawfords. *Hindu Bioethics for the Twenty First Century*. State University of New York Press, 2003.
7. Cromwell, *Ibid.*
8. Lipner. Julius J. *The Classical Hindu View on Abortion and the Moral Status of the Unborn in Coward*, Lipner, Young, p. 42.
9. *Ibid.*
10. Cromwell Crawford *op.cit.*
11. *Ibid.*
12. *Ency. op cit.*, p. 1146.
13. *Ibid.*

Chapter 22

Health : Positive Bioethical Concept underlying *Vinaya Pitaka* — *Buddhism*

Riddhi Chakravarty

Introduction

The negative concept of health[1] as *absence of disease* is the traditional medical view of health. As opposite to this, the positive concept of health came into existence after the Second World War with the World Health Organization (WHO). To meet the need of the individuals and health care systems, WHO has defined health in a holistic[2] manner. Health being a resource for living, the concept has found a prime place in bioethics.[3] As a bioethical concern, health related issues are : right to health, obligation to the maintenance of health, responsibility for the maintenance of health, obligation to the maintenance of health, responsibility for the maintenance of health, just and fair access to health and health care, etc.

In the Indian perspective of the relation between bioethics and health, the study of Buddhism and medicine hints that the concept of health in Buddhism adheres to the medical concept of health, whereas, literature review in depth suggests the existence of holistic model of health in Buddhism. The question then arises, is the holistic model propounded by WHO and Buddhism the same and similar ? Addressing this question, this chapter will first conceptualize health as a positive concept through the holistic model as propounded by WHO. Next, this chapter will explicate the concept of health as found in the text of *Vinaya Pitaka.* Then the conclusion will be drawn by arguing that while positive concept of health has been a recent bioethical concern, but Buddhism had propounded the concept much earlier, however, in an unlikely manner.

Section I

Health being an interdisciplinary issue of discussion from the last century, the Holisitc model came into light. Under this model health has been defined as a *state of sound mind, in a sound body, in a sound atmosphere, in a sound environment.* It implies that health is a multidimensional process involving the well-being of the whole person in the context of the surrounding environment. Within this model comes the 1948 WHO definition of health as a *state of complete physical, mental and social well-being and not merely the absence of disease or infirmity.* The model in this sense broadened the medical model perspective of health as the absence of disease and introduced the idea of 'positive health'.

Decades later, through the health promotion initiative, WHO has promoted the *Wellness Model,* and expanded the concept of health as *the extent to which an individual or group is able to realize aspirations and satisfy needs, to change or cope with the environment.* It explains the concept of *health as a resource for everyday life,* but *not the objective of living* (that can be achieved year later); it describes health as a *positive concept, as well as physical capabilities* (WHO, 1986). The model has further broadened the perspective of medical model by introducing the concept of quality of life (QOL) lived each day of which health is an essential component and has also assigned an intrinsic value on health.

The positive health as put forward by WHO conceptualizes

health is influenced by biological, psychological and also social factors. It implies the notion of perfect harmonization and function of mind and body. Introducing health in this way, the present author's claim is that although much has been discussed about Buddhism and health in relation to bioethics and medical ethics, but nothing exposes the actual nature of health as maintained by the Buddhist tradition. So, the next section tries to support the claim by referring to the Buddhist text of *Vinaya Pitaka.*

Section II

In relation to Buddhism and medicine, it can be mentioned that in *Suttanipata,* it is said that in order to attain *nirvana*, one should have certain indifferences. So it is said,

> "*aathabbanam supinam lakkhanam/no vidaha atho pi nakkattam/viruttam ca gabbhakaranam/tikiccham mamako na seveyya//*", (*Tuvattakasuttam,* 1927), that is, occasions as mentioned in *Atharva Veda, svapno, nimitta, nakshatra* one should not have involvement regarding these subjects; any followers of Buddha would not exercise the songs of animals and birds, causing impregnation, and also not the art of medicine. (*Silabhadra* 2002 : 147).

Thus on the one hand, while study of medicine has been prescribed as a prohibitory act, on the other hand, it is believed in Buddhism that voluntarily and compassionately helping a sick with the perceived susceptibility to reduce the severity of the disease is a virtue. Focusing this virtue aspect of the voluntary care giving, medicine gradually became an integral part of Buddhism[4], forming the earliest systematic exposition or medicine.[5]

One of the Buddhist texts containing such references of values of medicine is *vinaya pitaka.* The *Bhesaijya Skandhak* of the *Mahavagga* of *Vinaya Pitaka* discusses several diseases and their treatments through the words of Buddha. Thus it is mentioned that when there was a malnutrition and loss of appetite due to sickness of seasonal influenza among the *bhikhus* of the Jetavana of Anathpindaka (*Sravasti*), Bhagvan instructed to take ghee, butter, oil, honey and jaggery/molasses at the right moment and use them at the right time (*Vin.Pit. mahavagga* 6.1:211). Fats as foods being a requirement at that time for the *bhikhus* suffering from malnutrition, Gautama prescribed to take at the right time the oil cooked fresh fat of bear, fish, alligators, swine, and of asses and instructed to take them within one day, violation of which commits punishable offence (*dukata dosa*)(*ibid.*, 6. 3:212), Intake of raw meat and raw blood were also permitted whenever there was a requirement only (*ibid., 6.13:214)*[6]. But later on, in the context of sacrificing own flesh by Supriya, it is mentioned that whatever may be the situation; crises, drought, famine, etc., one is not supposed to take flesh of elephant, horse, snake, lion, tiger, panther, bear, and hyena (*tarakka*) (*ibid.*, 6.98-106:229). Thus, although flesh taking was considered in necessity but not unnecessarily out of grudge and only to meet the hunger.

As the popularity of Buddha and Buddhism rose, Buddha's medicinal prescriptions also gained importance. Simultaneously there were risk of criticisms and gossips of eating non-vegetarian food by the *bhikhus.* So Buddha said that in three cases non-vegetarian foods like fish and meat are pure; if one does not see it while eating, if one does not hear about it during intake of food, and if one does not suspect that it has been caught specially to be given to himself (*ibid.*, 6.110:241).

Besides prescribing the use of appetizer and flesh as foodstuffs, Buddha was also concerned of the usefulness of the foods of plant origin. While being at Jetavana among the *bhikhus* suffering from seasonal influenza, Gautama felt the need of taking medicinal roots by the suffering *bhikhus*. So he granted the permission to take medicinal roots like turmeric, ginger, orris, white orris, *atisa,* black hellebore, special *bhadramuktaa (nagarmotha)* and other roots of medicinal values which the *bhikhus* otherwise neglected (*op. cit.*, 6.5: 212).

Suffering from malnutrition requires vegetable and fruit extracts for fast recovery. So Buddha, prescribed taking of astringent decoctions of *neem, kutaj, patol, paggva, naktamaala* and other astringent roots, hard or soft, used for medicine or for imparting appetizing flavour to foods, which the sick *bhikhus* otherwise could not eat and discarded easily (*ibid.*, 6.6:212-213). Moreover, he also prescribed medicines made of different kinds of leaves like *neem, kutaja, patol, tulasi, kapasika,* and whatever other kinds which can be used both as medicines and appetizing flavours to food (*ibid.*, 6.7:213). Of fruits, he mentioned of *vidanga, pippali, mircha, harra, bahera, amal, gosthaphala,* and whatever other fruit medicines exist (*ibid.*,6.8:213). Besides these medicines, Gautama also felt the need of gum medicine for the ailing *bhikhus* of Jetavana. So he mentioned of partaking *hingu, hingu* lac, *sipatika, taka, takapatti, taka panni, sajjulasa* and others. (*ibid., 6.9:213).* Moreover, he also felt the need of medicines made of salt. So he mentioned taking of different kinds of salt : *samudrik, kala, sendha, vanaspatic, virala* and of other kinds. (*ibid.*, 6.10:213). Perhaps to beat the rough weather, to take precautionary measures from being dehydrated, different kinds of juices and salts were prescribed.

He is also said to have allowed application of medicinal to those who has itch, boils, discharge, ill smelling body and to those in ill health, the use of dry dung, clay and of clearing matter for keeping the skin free of dust and infections (*op.cit.*, 6.11:213). For boils only, Buddha prescribed lancet, decoctions of stringent herbs, sesamum salve, compress, oil for wounds, and fine rags for bandages (*ibid.*, 6.56:217). Along with boils, leprosy, consumption, and fit being prevailing diseases of the time, Buddha prescribed not sharing same utensils of food, clothes and other necessary things with the person infected with the diseases. This prescription was sort of a preventive measure against any kind of epidemic. Thus, besides permitting different nutritious and healthy diet for the *bhikhus* his concern was over ill health of the *bhikhus.*

For eye disease, uses of kajal, wick, and kajal container were also prescribed. Use of eye ointments and pastes were also permitted but while only suffering from eye disease (*Vin. Pit.*

Culavagga. 5.1.18:416). Use of perfumes made of sandalwood, *tagara,* black *anusari, katuya* and *bhaddamuttaka* were prescribed only when necessity springs up to grind up into ointments (*ibid.,* 6.14-25:215).

Moreover, taking medicines made of cow urine decoctions were prescribed for jaundice; anointing perfumes and aromatic drugs for skin diseases; and dung; urine, ashes, and clay-filth against snake bite. Decoction of dung was also prescribed as anemetic and poisons (*ibid.,* 6.66, 61-62:218).

During sickness, the patients require a care giver to take care of. In this regard, Buddha prescribed stay of care givers. (*ibid.,* 6.72:19).

For the maintenance of fitness, Buddha prescribed milk products like *kshiram, dadhi, takkam, nanvita, sappim* (*ibid.,* 6.11:245). Moreover, he is said to have prescribed keeping rice and different kinds of pulses with oneself, while making journey through rough terrains (*ibid.,* 6.116:246).

To check the seriousness of the disease, viewing of mirrors was also granted (*Vin. Pit. Culavagga* 5.16:416). Moreover, it was also instructed that going outside without carrying any water is punishable. (*ibid.,* 5.96:425). As the necessity of water was felt within the *viharas,* the permission of well was also granted (*ibid.,* 5.147-169:428-429). These prescriptions may be due to the dry weather condition of the area and also for the hygienic reasons.

For the maintenance of the germ-free environment, Buddha prescribed separate place for storing foodstuffs and cooking materials and mentioned four kinds of store rooms : one made of pillars. another for cows, third one for keeping foodstuffs and the fourth one of keeping other kinds of stuffs (*Vin. Pit. Mahavagga,* 113-114:242). There was prescriptions for keeping separate for medicines, and other stuffs (*Vin. Pit. Culavagga.,* 5.90:424).

As per Wilson (2004) "*Vinaya Pitaka* provides two forms of medical information : material and stories of treatments based on cases of diseases". While the above discussions are of material medica type, at the next portion will discuss the stories of treatments based on cases of diseases.

Once, *ayushman* Sariputra was said to be suffering from *kaidaha* (skin problem). He asked his friend Maudgalyana to bring him some lotus root and lotus stalk by eating which he can be completely cured of the problem (*Vin. Pit. Mahavagga.* 6.93-94:225). The story thus hints the medicinal use of the lotus plants. In the *culavagga* of the *Vinaya Pitaka*, the technique of how to take proper bath during normal body condition and also while having some skin problem is mentioned, along which it is also mentioned that violation of it causes *dukatta* crime (*Vin. Pit. Culavagga.* 5.11:415-416).

From the story of Gautama Buddha's wandering in Rajagriha, it is known that for the diseased person, Buddha prescribed molasses but for the persons without any disease, he prescribed juice made of molasses. This prescription again seemed to combat the dry weather of the particular region.

While taking invitation to Keniya Jatila's house; Buddha gave permission of only eight kinds of drinks of fruits : *amra jambu, coch, moch, madhu, angora, saluki,* and *farusak*, excepting the drinks of the vegetables. He is also said to prescribe partaking of edible fruits of all kinds and juices of all kinds except those of intoxicating qualities (*Vin. Pit. Mahavagga.* 118:247).

The disease of rheumatism was common at the time. Once, Pilindabaccho was suffering from it along with blistering feet. Buddha prescribed oil massage, hot water baths with some medicinal herbs being stuped in water. He is also said to have instructed letting of blood by a horn for intermittent ague and water treatment for blistering feet (*ibid.*, 6.41-57:216-218).

From the above discussion, it follows that Buddhism propounds to treat the patient after diagnosing the disease first (*glanapratyaya*) and then prescribing the application of medicine with the proper use *(bhaisajyadana)*. In this context. Buddhism follows the four noble truths as a 'pattern of pathology *(nidana)*'[7]. Hence, it can be said that Buddhism with its epidemiological study of medicine aims at the cure and prevention of the disease, at both the diagnosis and prognosis of the diseases.

Besides these prescriptions of medicines and diets, in *Vinaya Pitaka*, it is also said that Buddha had introduced rules among monks regarding rooms for urinals, urinal outlets, latrine chambers, and latrine outlets with proper measurements and also of water pipes for supplying water within the then form of toilet complex. He had also instructed to build wells within the *viharas* for keeping the complex neat, clean and hygienic. It is also said that some of these rules are also for common people. One of these includes that in a clean and green surrounding, so long one is fit and fine, one should not urinate and make free of other wastes hither and tither, in green areas and in water.[8] He thus tried to give knowledge of sanitary science at first to the monks and nuns and afterwards to the local common people outside the *viharas*.[9] Apart from the knowledge of hygiene, other message that he conveyed through these instructions is the message of proper housing which was introduced much later by WHO:

> Housing is intimately related to health. The structure, location, facilities, environment and uses of human shelter have a strong impact on the state of physical, mental, and social well-being. Poor housing conditions and uses may provide weak defenses against death, and injury or even increase vulnerability to them. Adequate and appropriate housing conditions, on the other hand, not only protect people against health hazards but also help to promote robust physical health, economic productivity, psychological well-being and social vigour (WHO, 1989).

Summarizing the section it can be said that like World Health Organization, Buddhism had also propounded the holistic concept of health. Next section describes whether the two traditions have any similarity in conceptualizing health or not.

Conclusion

The earlier section suggests that Sakyamuni's view of the healing arts was eminently practical and therapeutic. But the goals of this therapeutic treatment do not end in maintaining perfect health only.

It focuses on the person as a whole. Given the difficulty of maintaining health in severe weather conditions like drought, poverty, famine, and hunger, his pragmatic approach included simple, easy available resources with insistence on proper hygiene and better sanitary conditions. In addition, it can be said that Buddha focused above all to the discipline of making these as regular habit, for which it is mentioned repeatedly that disobeying rules and restrictions will cause *dukkata dosa.*

With this regular practice of simple and balanced standard of living, Buddhism is said to ask the monks to bring a complete harmony in between mind and body. Thus, Buddhism propounds the concept of positive health, the optimal condition of health, which can be achieved only when mind and body function are well and interact together as one, amidst the favourable condition. Moreover, as Keown (2001, 4) point out the following Birnbaum that indisposition and ill health weaken the mind and shift the focus of meditation. And so securing healthy physical status and maintaining good health was a prerequisite for the disciplined monastic life. In addition it can also be said that medicine seemed to be a practice of monastic life because, as Zysk (Keown, 2001) points out that with the monks as the healers and monatic structures as the infirmaries and hospices, monasteries extend the support to the common people beyond its boundary.

Hence, it can be said that like Kant, Gautama Buddha also propounded that Supreme Good can be attained by physical Good, that is, well-being and moral Good, that is, well-doing. *Bhikhus,* were prescribed to follow the rules of taking simple food, proper bath, and living in hygienic housing, etc., to discipline their lives as a healthy being. By voluntarily taking care of the sick[10], they were habituated to well doing. Combination of both the well-being and well-doing were prescribed to have the light of enlightenment on them[11]. In this sense, as opposite to the assignment of intrinsic value to the holistic view of health by WHO, Buddhism following *Vinaya Pitaka,* prescribes holistic and teleonomic (purposeful) view of health with simple diet, better living conditions and assigns an instrumental value to health along with the personal responsibility and obligation[12] to maintain one's own health and of others too.

This perspective of health in Buddhism can be said to reflect the recent concern of bioethics, where health is considered as the critical concept and special Good for (i) directly affecting person's well-being and (ii) for being a prerequisite to a person's functioning as an agent to pursue different goals and projects in life that one values (Anand, 2004). Thus while the trend of bioethics and its concern of health has been a recent emergence, but the text of *Vinaya Ptaka* suggests that Buddhism has advanced all these a long time back and is inherent in the tradition of Buddhism, which when followed properly can save people from certain health hazards.

NOTES

1. Anand, Sudhir, 2004. The Concern for Equity in Health. In *Public Health, Ethics, and Equity,* New Delhi: Oxford University Press.
2. Bapat, P.V. (1924). 1990. *The Sutta-Nipata. Bibliotheca* Indo-Buddhica No. 75:267, Delhi: Sri Satguru Publication.
3. Bhikku Silabhadra. 2002. *Sutta Nipata.* Kolkata: Maha Bodhi Book Agency.
4. Callahan, Daniel and Bruce Jennings. 2002. Ethics and Public Health: Forging a Strong Relationship. In *American Journal of Public Health,* No. 2 (92):169-176.
5. Chattopadhayay, Debiprasad, 1977. *Science and Society in Ancient India,* 323-341, Calcutta: Research India Publications.
6. Daniels, Norman, 2008. Just *Health, Meeting Health Needs Fairly.* New York: Combridge University Press.
7. Gorovitz, Samuel. 1978. Health as an Obligation in. Warren T. Reich ed. *Encyclopedia of Bioethics,* vol. 607-609, New York: The Free Press.
8. Immanuel Kant. (1930). 1979. *Lecture On Ethics,* Trans. Louis Infield, Great Britan: Methuen & Co. Ltd.
9. Keown, Damien. (1995) 2001. Buddhism and Bioethics, London: Palgrave Publishers Limited.
10. ——., and J.Hughes. 1995. Buddhism And Medical Ethics: A Bibliographic Introduction. In *Journal of Buddhist Ethics.* Volume 2:105-124.

http://www.buddhistethics.org/2/hughes.txt. (Accessed on 24 June, 2009).

11. Khusf, George. 2004. *Handbook of Bioethics: Taking Stock of the Field from a Philosophical Perspective,* Netherlands: Kluwer Academic Publisher, Springer, ISBN 142018703, 9781402018701
12. McGee, Glen, (1999) 2003. Pragmatic Method and Bioethics in Pragmatic Bioethics ed. Glen McGee, Masachusetts: MIT Press.
13. Nakamura, Hajime. 1978, Buddhism in. Warren T. Reich ed. *Encyclopedia of Bioethics,* vol 1: 134-138, New York: The Free Press.
14. Park, K. (1970). 2005. Park's Textbook of Preventive and Social Medicine, Jabalpur: Banarsidas Bhanot Publishers.
15. Parsons, Talcott. 1978. A Sociological and Action Perspective. In *Health and Disease,* Encyclopedia of Bioethics. ed. W.t.Reich, vol. 2: 590-599.
16. Potter, Van Rensselaer. 1971 *Bioethics, Bridge to the Future.* Englewood Cliffs, N.J: Prentice-Hall, Inc.
17. Risse, Guenter B.1978. History of the Concepts. In Health and Disease, *Encyclopedia of Bioethics.* ed. W.T. Reich, vol 2: 579-585.
18. Sanskritayan, Rahul 1934. *Vinaya Pitaka.* Taiwan: The Corporate Body of the Buddha Educational Foundation.
19. Sharma, P.V. (Ed.) 1992. Medicine in Buddhist and Jaina Traditions. *In History of Medicine in India.* New Delhi: Indian National Science Academy.
20. Wilson, Liz., 2004, Perspectives On The Body in *Encyclopedia of Buddhism, Vol* 1:63-66, ed. Robert E. Buswell, U.S.A. : MacMillan Reference.
21. WHO 1989. *Health Principles of Housing* Geneva.
22. Zysk, Kenneth G. 2004. Medicines *In Encyclopedia of Buddhism,* ed. Robert E. Buswell, Vol. 2:518-519, U.S.A.: MacMillan Reference.

Index